Praise for *Helping Mothers, Helping Babies*

"Dr. Leslie Costello uses her vast experience as a clinician working with perinatal women to provide a thorough and thoughtful book. She makes a theoretically solid and impassioned plea to therapists, arguing for a somatic approach to healing. Leslie points out that, 'Unmet feelings arise in mothers of new babies . . . When a baby is demanding everything from you, the blank spots in your own emotional experience become painful chasms that you cannot even describe.' A rich array of somatic techniques is provided for therapists to try and to use with their clients. Here is her argument for somatic work with the abdomen. 'Culturally, we have a lot of unrealistic expectations for our midsections . . . Most people have bellies that are overly tight and held-in or are loose and uncontained because of weak muscles. People who have recently given birth have bellies that have been through a lot and need a lot of love.'

The clinical case vignettes punched me in the heart! For example, a new mother had a baby whose crying reminded the mother of her abusive ex-husband. Leslie's work with this client reveals what she preaches in the book—her use of compassionate inquiry and how she follows the body to provide a somatic shift that brings new insights to the client.

In the summary, Leslie writes, 'Helping women to take the mantle of maternal identity in a way that genuinely honors the individual is significant . . . Perinatal therapists keep our eyes firmly on the mother. She is the locus of our work, and yet there is an element of the future in perinatal therapy that can make it even more meaningful.' And that future involves all of us. A woman who feels grounded in her body, vital, and able to manage her new role as a mother creates a kind of peace that spreads from her home and radiates out to the whole society."

— **Vincentia Schroeter, PhD** Author of *Communication Breakthrough: How Brain Science and Listening to Body Cues Can Transform Your Relationships* (2018) and *Baby Quest* (forthcoming). Co-author: *Bend Into Shape: Techniques for Bioenergetic Therapists* (2011)

"*Helping Mothers, Helping Babies* is a vital contribution to the emerging and direly needed field of somatically informed perinatal mental health. Costello brings a depth of clinical wisdom, research, and embodied understanding to the realities of the perinatal journey—offering a much-needed shift from a 'baby-first' lens to a mother-centered, integrative approach. With clarity and compassion, she weaves somatic interventions into the therapeutic process, making this book an invaluable resource for clinicians seeking to support mothers in their full complexity. Costello's work resonates deeply with the timely emphasis on maternal embodied healing as foundational to perinatal care on both individual, family, and community levels. This book is a must-read for any practitioner committed to bridging the gap between psychology and the lived, felt experience of the maternal body."

— **Helena Vissing, PsyD, SEP, PMH-C**, Associate Professor at CIIS and author of *Somatic Maternal Healing: Psychodynamic* and *Somatic Trauma Treatment for Perinatal Mental Health*

"This beautifully written and deeply informative book is infused with palpable compassion and expertise borne of Dr. Costello's decades of work with the perinatal population. Throughout this practical and accessible guide, the author seamlessly integrates somatic, body-based approaches with relatable vignettes and insights from decades of experience as a perinatal therapist. In creating this guide for clinicians and other helping professionals in the perinatal sphere, Dr. Costello continues to offer invaluable support for mothers navigating the profound physical, emotional, and psychological shifts of motherhood.

Filled with immediately usable, intuitive somatic tools, this guide is grounded in a deep understanding of trauma-informed care. It presents accessible, research-backed techniques that feel natural and are proven to be highly effective in clinical practice. The book itself is thoughtfully structured, making it easy to navigate and integrate into therapy sessions.

Insightful, empowering, and deeply practical, this book is an invaluable resource for any clinician committed to supporting mothers in a holistic, embodied way. An essential addition to every therapist's bookshelf!"

— **Jaimee Folkins, MEd, CCC, LCT, PMH-C**, owner and psychotherapist at Balanced Beginnings Counselling Therapy

"In this valuable book, Leslie thoroughly describes the challenges perinatal women encounter and offers a toolkit of somatic resources to help them. The book incorporates rich case examples, clear explanations of the theory and techniques of bioenergetic therapy, and a guide to deepening self-awareness and psychotherapy practice. I highly recommend it to therapists and their perinatal clients."

— **Laurie Ure, LICSW**, Certified Bioenergetic Therapist, Faculty Member, International Institute for Bioenergetic Analysis

"Therapists know that healing is a continuous process—not only for clients but for themselves as well. In *Helping Mothers, Helping Babies*, Dr. Leslie Costello offers a well-researched, practical guide to integrating somatic therapy into work with birthing individuals. This book is an essential resource for therapists supporting perinatal clients, providing valuable insights and concrete exercises to navigate the complexities of pregnancy, postpartum transitions, and perinatal mood disorders. A must-read for mental health professionals dedicated to deepening their practice and enhancing care for growing families."

— **Sarah Branson, CNM, MSN**

A MANUAL FOR THERAPISTS

HELPING MOTHERS, HELPING BABIES

Somatic Perinatal Psychotherapy

LESLIE ANN COSTELLO, PhD

Devon Station Books

HELPING MOTHERS, HELPING BABIES

To request permission, contact the publisher at Devonstationbooks@gmail.com
Paperback: 978-1-7390170-5-7
First paperback edition March 2025
E-book: 978-1-7390170-6-4

Illustrations by Maggie Vicknair
Cover design by Kam Bains
Editing by Nanette Littlestone
Interior design by Peter Hildebrandt

Nothing in this book constitutes medical care or a substitute for medical care. Use exercises with caution and at your own risk.

Devon Station Books
242 Neill Street
Fredericton, NB, CA
Devonstationbooks.com

Dedication

Writing is a solitary endeavour, but the process invokes many people. In working on this book, I sat with memories of my clients and supervisees and my hopes for future readers.

I dedicate this book to the clients who have trained me, their therapist, to listen deeply and support firmly while they get on with the courageous work of becoming themselves. I continue to hold their stories of longing, loss, and discovery as sacred offerings, ever more grateful for their trust. The suffering and healing in my therapy room has shaped me and shaped this volume.

It is also dedicated to therapists. As I wrote, I held the image of you, the therapist, using these tools and ideas to shape your own theory and practice. In addition to holding the space for client experiences, therapists hold an optimistic image of the future. You hold the image of integration, clarity, and healing that a client cannot yet visualize for herself. If there is a magic in therapy, your capacity to create hope could be it.

My deep desire is for this book to help you imagine and create the path forward.

Contents

Exercises/Case Examples

About the Author

Leslie Ann Costello, PhD, is a psychologist and bioenergetic therapist. After a career as a preschool teacher, she studied developmental psychology at George Mason University in Fairfax, Virginia. Study, research, and teaching in infant mental health ultimately led her to study maternal mental health, after professional encounters with pregnancy and infant loss. As a freshly minted PhD, she landed in a grant-funded prenatal clinic in Louisiana, soaking up experiences that shaped the trajectory of her thirty-year career as professor, therapist, trainer, and supervisor. Certified in bioenergetic analysis, in perinatal mental health, and trained in Circle of Security Parenting and EMDR, she brings a variety of perspectives to bear on her topic.

As a speaker and workshop leader, Leslie has shared her experiences with public health nurses, counselors and psychotherapists, community support workers, somatic therapists, and parents. In leading groups, she strives to create spaces for others to share their voices and strengthen the web of connections that support all of us in doing the work that matters.

Grace Notes (Gratitude)

I never really know what to say in these moments. My heart overflows with appreciation for the support I've received in the process of creating this book, and when I'm overcome with feeling, my words stutter.

But I can take a breath and try again. None of the work I've done has been on my own: I have been blessed with support and encouragement since graduate school. Writing this book started with study and practice, teaching, training, conversations with peers—wine included when possible—and ultimately an idea that I might have something to share. That idea turned into articles about bioenergetics and perinatal psychotherapy, and my original concept for the book was to compile those articles. Easy peasy!

As it turns out, a book is not just a compilation; it needs an identity and a life of its own. The metaphor of birth might be cliché, but it is also apt. This one has been years in the writing but many more years in practice and conceptualization.

I can't properly thank everyone who contributed to my thinking around these topics. Vincentia Schroeter's coaching helped me consider my intended reader as well as see myself as a writer. Early readers and commenters included Susan Kanor, Carole Melnick, Bethany Doyle, Ailsa Keppie, and Adela Gorodzinsky.

Later readers included Laurie Ure, Vincentia Schroeter, Helena Vissing, Meri Levy, Sarah Branson, Jaimee Folkins, and Theresa Gil. Many thanks for your time and your thoughtful reflection.

My gratitude extends to the wonderful bioenergetic trainees who allowed me to practice teaching somatic skills in vivo, to the therapists willing to meet to discuss my twin passions of infant mental health and maternal mental health, and to those who have invited me into their offices and living rooms to explore the somatic tools we can bring to bear in psychotherapy.

My beloved partner in life, Dan Beaudette, has been a supporter of this process from the beginning and has tolerated my waffling with equanimity. He's held a clear vision of completion. His encouragement has been no small matter in getting the book into readers' hands.

Prologue

Childbearing is a time of physical, social, psychic, and spiritual changes for the mother and the people close to her. Birth is a liminal moment, when the mother and baby are poised between worlds. Crossing that threshold changes everything. While the drama of the expulsion from intrauterine life to the outside world is obvious, the birthing woman changes in ways that are no less profound.

Under ideal circumstances, both infant and mother will transition relatively smoothly, though severe postpartum reactions have been recorded for centuries. Caring for a newborn is hard work for a mother, even with excellent support, especially when she is also recovering from pregnancy and childbirth. In many cases, the transition into motherhood is fraught, and women face more challenges than their resources can tolerate.

Modern expectations of women don't include accommodation for pregnancy or a prolonged adjustment period after the baby is born. Social roles continue, with the addition of a new baby, potentially making postpartum life hard to navigate. The advent of extreme social sharing on networks has resulted in a wider awareness and, we hope, acceptance of challenges in the perinatal period.

I use the term "perinatal" to include fertility struggles, pregnancy, childbirth and the first postpartum year, for both the mother and infant. In her excellent book *Somatic Maternal Healing*, my colleague Helena Vissing makes the point that "perinatal therapy" has become associated with prenatal and infant experiences of a person as a fetus and infant, thus shifting the orientation away from the mother-baby dyad. She has chosen to refer to "maternal healing" to focus on the mother. Vissing's decision highlights a common problem: maternal struggles often are ignored in favor of overwhelming attention to the baby. This occurs not only in social situations but also in helping relationships. Even therapists can inadvertently reinforce mothers' tendencies to downplay their suffering when looking through a "baby first" lens. This book assumes "mother first," while recognizing that the mother's well-being makes a difference to children and partners.

In this volume, I use "perinatal" because of the widespread application to diagnosis of maternal mental health issues that occur proximate to the childbearing year. In fact, clinicians use shorthand (PMADs) to refer to Perinatal Mood and Anxiety Disorders. These disorders include depression, generalized anxiety, obsessive-compulsive disorder, panic, and trauma-related disorders as they connect with childbearing.

We all have our implicit biases and unarticulated expectations. My original training as a developmental psychologist predisposed me to think of the infant first. However, to do our best work for mothers we have to be oriented to helping them for their own sake. At the same time, mothers' recent and concurrent reproductive experiences are germane. Specialized training for therapists makes a difference, not least because it helps us locate, articulate, and separate from our biases.

It is hard to overstate the urgency of the perinatal situation. PMADs and postpartum stress in general can be disabling. At the very least, they result in suffering, a grave contrast to the romanticized social image of mothering an infant. The prevalence of PMADs is not trivial, and there is clear evidence of an increase during and after the pandemic of 2020–2022, when lockdowns imposed social isolation and limited opportunities for family support.

The dynamic nature of early parenting means we cannot allow mothers to languish on waiting lists. They need effective help immediately. Too often, mothers' deep desperation can go unnoticed. Maternal suicide is the largest contributor to maternal mortality (see Chin et al. 2022). Obviously, women who are struggling need effective support now.

Even in the "mother first" model, there is also a baby, and maybe other children, to consider. Most mothers provide the majority of caregiving context for newborns through the first year of life, and as such, they are the primary source of input to a new brain that's laying down and pruning lifetime connections. While it is patently unhelpful to remind a struggling woman of this responsibility, professionals hold this broader context in mind. When you work to support women in this period, you are making an impact beyond the individual. Helping parents is a real, concrete way of making the future better.

As awareness grows, resources follow. The increasing public awareness of challenges of pregnancy and postpartum has resulted in the development of perinatal psychotherapy—therapy with mothers—as a subspeciality complete with available education, training, and certification. In the thirty years I've been engaged with this work, perinatal mental health work—including case management, counseling, psychotherapy, and psychiatry—has blossomed in response to increasing need.

Who chooses this specialty for therapy? We are drawn to the work in different ways and from different fields—social work, counseling, nursing, psychology. My interest was piqued by doing research with bereaved families and, in an unusual juxtaposition, toddler attachment. Many others bring personal experience with fertility issues, birth trauma, or PMADs. The experience of recovery can fuel a desire to help others, and in general, the field is full of people who are generous with ideas and resources.

Collaboration makes the most of our different backgrounds and orientations. When perinatal therapists get together, even online, and share strengths, there's a rich exchange of ideas and inquiry. The pandemic brought many new things, including a rich experience of online learning.

This book supports you in bringing the body explicitly into your work with perinatal clients. While therapists often offer suggestions around sleep, nutrition, and exercise, actual somatic interventions during the session are less common.

However, they are well suited to perinatal clients, who are busy, exhausted, and suffering. These interventions are brief, experiential, and easy to use at home. They offer rapid relief from common complaints without requiring deep probing about feelings. Somatic interventions have lasting benefits, including increased self-acceptance, interpersonal connection, emotion regulation, and high-quality parenting.

The practices in this book support any of the therapy models you already use, but they are more than an add-on. A tenet of somatic practice is to experience every exercise before trying it with clients. Using the tools yourself gives you access to your own body wisdom, as well as support for holding

---

Somatic interventions

- Are brief & experiential
- Offer rapid relief
- Don't probe deeply into feelings
- Have lasting benefits

---

your clients' trauma, releasing any distress you might be holding for the client and accessing your pleasure and joy.

Each exercise includes directions for personal practice along with specific instructions for introducing exercises to clients. I've included case examples so you can see how a somatic intervention might be a natural part of a session. Case examples are created from composite clients, rather than representing a particular individual.

Some of the terminology may be unfamiliar, so I have included a glossary.

The exercises in this book are not a substitute for medical or psychological care.

Anyone doing somatic work needs to consider their own needs for adaptation, change or modification. For some people, even mild exercise should not be attempted without consultation with a medical practitioner. Use your discretion, clinical judgment, and your self-knowledge in choosing how to use this book.

Introduction

The transition to parenthood can be stressful, and people's responses vary. The physical changes in pregnancy and birth, sleep deprivation, brain fog, and the pressing social, financial, and identity issues are challenging for anyone. If a person is already stressed or in distress, these issues can be powerfully destabilizing.

> Becoming a happier mother means everything to women who are struggling. It can mean a lifetime of difference for their children.

Like most life transitions, the perinatal time is one of opportunity and challenge. When a person finds fertility, pregnancy, postpartum or motherhood especially difficult, distress can bring about a cascade of somatic, psychological, and psychosocial effects.

Our clients' bodies are the common ground for the two threads of somatic psychotherapy and perinatal mental health. The perinatal psychological experience is created from somatic experience. Sex, fertility, pregnancy, birth, and lactation are clearly body experiences. Less obvious, perhaps, is the body-ness of emotion, autonomic arousal, attention, memory, and relating. Our culture prioritizes mental activity, often ignoring direct experience, so our feelings, excitement or agitation, interests, and relationships are mediated by our thinking about them. In North American culture, even in psychotherapy, it is more common to think about and discuss feelings than it is to feel and express them.

Talking about how you feel isn't the same as feeling; it is one step removed from the experience. Somatic interventions focus on the here-and-now body experience, giving access to the everyday reality that underlies mental processing. Your somatic experience is a continuous flow, while your thinking is commentary. The foundation of experience is in the body, and changes there percolate upward to create mental changes.

Childbirth and caring for a newborn are life-changing events. Even when things are smooth, there is upheaval, resulting in some uncomfortable feelings and thoughts. Reducing those symptoms helps a woman adjust to her new role as a parent. Depending on her support network and personal resources, she might manage well. If she does come for help, somatic intervention—using breathing and attention to ease anxious symptoms—plus psychoeducation about perinatal distress, development of a stress-management plan, and social support might be sufficient, and if not, they still may be a good starting point.

Other mothers need more. Women with prior depression, anxiety, or a history of trauma may find that the chasm opened by the stress of the perinatal period is deep and wide. Rather than sensing the earth shake under her, she feels like her world is coming completely apart, with no solid ground anywhere, and she can barely recognize herself in the chaos (see Beck et al. 2013 for the earthquake analogy).

At the same time she's falling apart, the world denies her lived experience. She is bombarded with messages about how happy she should be, how wonderful her life is, and how precious it is to be a mother. The profound disconnection between her experience and social expectations contributes to the feeling of being unmoored in a hurricane. Now, when she feels least capable, she has a helpless baby to care for. No wonder she's struggling.

Therapy alleviates this desperate struggle. In therapy, she can set her burden down and be cared for, at least for an hour. During this time, her feelings matter and there might be hope for a better future. This is an opportunity for therapeutic change.

As a therapist, you have a small window in which to do this work. Demands on her resources as a new mother mean that she has limited time and energy. Therefore, focus on the here-and-now, helping her with immediate needs. Therapists also hold a long view. Short-term intervention may fuel long-term changes. Feeling better now helps her take better care of the baby. Although therapy in the perinatal period is primarily for the mother, it benefits the baby.

How to use this book

I've organized the book to be practical and easy to use. Chapters 1–4 describe perinatal development, perinatal therapy, and why and how to use somatic methods. Chapters 5–7 offer detailed preparation for doing the somatic work, identifying the skills that you will bring to your personal somatic explorations as well as your work with clients. Chapters 8–15 include exercises that you will explore personally before taking them into therapy. Chapter 15 has somatic interventions for you, the therapist, to avoid burnout.

There are sidebars with additional information. Exercises and case examples are identified in the Table of Contents. Cited sources are in the Bibliography, along with other helpful Resources.

Even though you'd probably rather skim the exercises, please practice them. There is no substitute for your own direct experience, because that's where your uniqueness arises. You'll find out more about yourself. I suggest you keep notes while you do the exercises. Jot down your impressions, how your body responds, what draws your attention, what memories arise while doing the movements. Doing the work yourself helps you explore with clients. The exercises are brief and can bring new insights. You're much more likely to introduce them to clients if you have explored them yourself.

There's a companion journal available to hold your notes and personal jottings. You'll find the link to this free download in the Resources section.

About bioenergetic analysis

Bioenergetic analysis is the name for an active, experiential, present-based psychotherapy. It offers a wholistic consideration of the mother in her context, including her developmental context and guidelines about interventions. It incorporates contemporary knowledge of trauma, neuroscience, and relational aspects of therapy.

Bio, as devotees familiarly call it, has been around for a long time, since the mid-twentieth century. Developed by Dr. Alexander Lowen, it is a comprehensive theory with psychoanalytic underpinnings. I trained in bio over an eight-year period, well into my career as a psychologist. The somatic orientation felt like home to me, and my own bio, undertaken as an essential part of training, changed my life in measurable ways.

There are other forms of body-oriented psychotherapy. They come from different schools of thought, and have different language, but they all work with the human body. You'll see many commonalities among body-oriented psychotherapies, as well as places of divergence.

While spokespeople and theorists articulate their distinctions, therapists who are working daily with clients typically do a lot of cross-pollinating, training in varied orientation and reading widely. I encourage you to dig around in literature from all the somatic models, as you're likely to find something useful and interesting in each.

A note about the orienting position

The standing exercises all begin from the "orienting position." The position is this: stand on the floor, feet under your hips, knees soft, head balanced comfortably on top of your spine, and eyes open. From here, you can orient to the room and any available stimulation—sounds, smells, sights. You can also orient to your own body, feeling how you are present in the space. Take the orienting position and check in.

A note about language

Perinatal work has focused largely on people who identify as women, and as such, our language may inadvertently leave out people who do not identify as women or mothers but who experience pregnancy, birth, and parenting. The work in these pages is applicable to all birthing persons, regardless of how they identify, and my use of language (most generally used by woman-identifying people) is not meant to exclude but reflects the experience of the majority of perinatal clients. I regret any discomfort that may arise out of my decision.

CHAPTER 1

Perinatal Mental Health and Body-Based Therapy

Perinatal mental health

We know, often implicitly, what can affect a person in the perinatal period. Making our implicit assumptions explicit gives a solid, reliable rationale for what we do in therapy. Putting together information, knowledge, and experiences constructs a framework or working model to understand what happens in perinatal development and what can go wrong.

How a woman proceeds through childbearing is affected by a myriad of variables. Generally, we tend to see clusters of risk and protective factors for PMADs falling into broad categories. These are social support and challenges, personal health and mental health history, and issues of identity, such as orientation to childbearing and child-rearing. Those broad categories don't do much to tell us about an individual client, but they can help us to understand where some of her stressors arise. We can keep these risk and protective factors in mind as we meet our client. Let's consider how that might work on an initial visit.

The above categories are part of my "working model" of perinatal functioning, but I don't necessarily ask about them. Instead, I assume she needs help immediately with some aspect of her functioning, so we begin with the here and now. While I listen and watch, I generate some ideas (hypotheses) based on those factors above. Without asking too many questions, I listen hard. Answers can come without a question being asked.

How is she doing? What is the biggest problem facing her? What are her current stressors and current ways to care for herself? How are sleep, nutrition, and healing from the pregnancy and birth? How are her relationships with her partner, other children, her family, and, of course, the baby? Is she able to enjoy anything?

Following threads from her answers, I'll ask about her birth experience, her pregnancy history, her mental health history. As needed, I inquire about her history of family and personal stress and who has been most helpful to her in her life (attachment history). All the time, I'm slotting information into my model of risk and protective factors, trying to understand what's operating here.

Social support and challenges to social support

As a therapist, I am deeply interested in my client's inner life—her experience. I want to know where she feels support and where it's lacking, from her perspective. I check on how things are with the partner, with her mother (and other family members), other children, her friends. Does she have support from a church or social network?

Personal health and mental health history

A pre-existing mental health diagnosis may be predictive of a PMAD. Health problems, either pre-dating pregnancy or resulting from pregnancy or birth, are important to keep in mind.

Orientation to childbearing and child-rearing

Women who chose to get pregnant, who had good support throughout pregnancy and birth, and who have wanted to become mothers are often shocked when things do not go smoothly. Mothers who were thrust into this new life without their full participation may be less shocked but also have fewer resources. Knowing something about the client's trajectory of acceptance across pregnancy, birth, and parenting can be helpful.

This assessment process may take several sessions, during which I'm building my relationship with her by listening hard for emotional content, reflecting and supporting her in her feelings, and giving her time and space to tell me what she wants to tell, as well as helping her to notice her body experience and including that in her self-narrative.

Our working model draws from a wide and deep understanding of the course of maternal identity, the effects of fertility challenges, the influences of prior mental health history on current functioning, and on and on. Many readers will also need the skills to make formal diagnoses, which are outside the scope of this volume. I've included a Resources section in the back of the book with helpful publications and contacts.

Perinatal distress

When a woman arrives in your office for help in the perinatal period, it is safe to make some assumptions.

First, it has taken a lot to get her to you. She has already tried everything she can imagine. Her contact with you is delicate and precious. You may be her last hope.

Next, she needs support, though she might not be able to define how it might look or feel. Your strong, clear message that you can be available for her with all her struggles is support. You provide her a place to be herself, with all her experiences.

You can assume she needs to be heard, including things she cannot talk about. Even the silence has meaning. She needs you to hear her suffering without offering judgment or advice, only support. This can be hard to remember, especially when you have some very useful advice to impart. Wait. Don't do it yet. Listen.

She's in defense mode. She won't necessarily be defensive with you, but know her defenses have been activated while trying to escape her symptoms. She's been trying to cope, but coping becomes defensive when initial efforts fail. Most people don't have great skills at climbing out of a hole, like depression or anxiety. The usual tactics don't work when all the ground rules have changed, as happens in the perinatal period. Defenses help people to feel safe under difficult circumstances, but they can also get in the way of healing.

Common defenses in perinatal distress

How many of these do you see in your clientele?

Isolation. Your client stays away from people and doesn't discuss her feelings. Through isolation, she can pretend that everything is okay and avoid her frightening thoughts. She may avoid talking to her partner, her doctor, or anyone who might be able to help her. She thinks she's fooling everyone, but the one she most wants to fool is herself.

Overwork. She may work excessively hard to be a "good mother." Overwork can take the form of insisting that only she can take care of the baby, obsessive cleaning, pumping more than the baby needs, or a dozen other things. It can include taking millions of pictures and posting them to social media. It can be a manifestation of OCD or simply a coping mechanism taken to an extreme.

Anger/irritability. Is she uncharacteristically angry? She projects feeling bad through her irritation and frustration onto anyone close, most often her partner. Rage is particularly frightening. Many clients are relieved to hear that these emotional storms are symptoms rather than a change in personality.

Dismissing. Does she dismiss or deny? She may assume that feeling terrible is part of being a mother, or that if she can pretend everything is fine, it really will be fine. She might refuse to acknowledge that anything is wrong, when everyone around her can see that there is something deeply amiss.

Self-criticism. Many clients are harsh with themselves. Oddly, self-criticism is a way to escape painful feelings. The mental activity of criticizing herself keeps her from feeling the fear coursing through her body. Listing all the things that are wrong with her can distract from feeling desperately alone and so tired she could die. Making an internal list of things to do better or to do immediately keeps her from feeling whatever scary feelings arise.

Somatically oriented therapists will also note the messages from her body. A focus on her physical well-being can keep her distracted too. There is more about how to do this in Chapters 5 and 7.

How defenses hurt

When someone's defense is to become highly self-critical, they suffer from the defense itself. When the defense is to become compulsive about safety or cleanliness, that creates suffering too. The defense can be harder to live with than just experiencing the emotion.

Why would we do such a thing? It's because the defense was created during a period in which it was needed for survival, either psychological survival or, in some cases, physical survival.

Defenses get activated when a new baby arrives on the scene. The life-or-death fragility of this demanding newborn is new. Parents pull out the survival strategies from their own early lives to help in this new situation, but many old defenses are useless or damaging in the present.

Defenses aren't inherently bad. They can be useful when they help us to navigate difficult patches. Defenses work until they stop working, but parents can get caught in patterns that prevent or delay them from getting help.

When your client can no longer deny how bad she feels, or when her family intervenes, it is because her defenses aren't working. If she hasn't seen her family physician, you can suggest a checkup. Get permission to communicate with the doctor, in any case.

Postpartum crisis

Most postpartum struggles are extremely difficult, but some are crises that need intervention. If your client has suicidal thoughts with a plan, and you cannot be sure she won't enact it, you must send her to emergency services immediately. If she has psychotic symptoms that are ego-syntonic (she doesn't see anything unusual about them), she needs medical assistance. If she feels unsafe, support her to seek emergency services. This is where you call in the family, and perhaps the police, to help support her to safety.

Please also note that "scary thoughts" that frighten the client—about hurting the baby, or the baby getting hurt, or the mother getting hurt—are common and not an indication of intention or likelihood of taking this action. Making this distinction can be challenging and is one of the reasons we strongly recommend that therapists working with this population obtain specialized training.

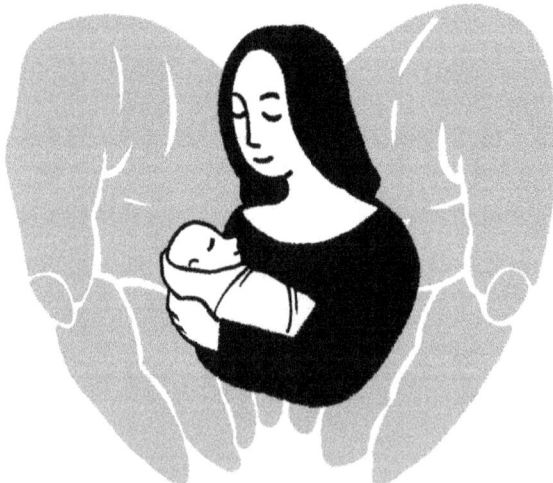

Somatic (body-based) psychotherapy

Many therapy models skip the body entirely. Even though your clients walk into your office in a body, the physical is not only in the back seat but often ignored. The fact that the brain, where we popularly believe our minds to be housed, is incontrovertibly part of the body suggests that bypassing somatic experience is shortsighted at best.

All of us have bodies, and our body experiences are our lives. Talk therapy is oriented to thinking and behavior, but both of those activities require a body. Mental state is a function of physical state, though it also exerts an influence on physical state. Most obviously, reproductive issues arise from the body experiences of the client.

New approaches integrate the body into therapeutic work, via mindfulness, stress management, or explicit focus on autonomic reactivity. Our current understanding of trauma, for example, has helped mainstream psychotherapy to grasp that the body is not just a vessel for the mind but the place where the person experiences her life. Psychology and physiology are not opposite; in fact, they are pretty much the same thing, observed through different lenses.

Adding the body to our working model of perinatal development

Our somatically informed working model includes the inherent wisdom of the body. Our body experiences form the basis of thoughts and feelings, including disturbing ones. When someone is lost in frightening thoughts, just attending directly to the body for a few minutes can bring a bit of relief. All forms of relaxation start with attention to the body, often in the form of noticing the breath. Shifts in the body generate shifts in the psyche and the emotional life.

Bodies are self-healing. When you break a leg, the surgeon sets the bone, but the body heals itself. This is also true for issues of emotional distress. The person, or at least her body, knows how to heal. She will heal if the obstacles are removed. In therapy, we deconstruct those obstacles to make space for being with difficult feelings. Just being with feelings often "heals," allowing the person to turn attention elsewhere rather than focus on avoiding the emotion.

Bodies are continually in resonance with other bodies. The therapist's body is present in the session too. You are relating to your client and your body; your somatic self is relating to her somatic self. This is a continuous, generally unconscious, process that happens across relationships. Agitated babies who are too young to self-regulate their arousal are calmed by a parent's easy unruffled response. Without thinking about it, people share their children's excitement or ease a partner's distress. Therapists pay close attention to their own somatic experiences in therapy, noting how their process interacts with their clients' process.

Remembering that the body has its own wisdom is a guide, especially useful to therapists when we don't know what to do next. (Yes, we all have those moments in session!) Knowing our presence is vitally important gives value to moments of connection with our client—the moments in which we sit in relationship with her, sharing in her experience, creating space for whatever she is feeling.

Understanding the body as self-healing allows us to step away from prescriptive strategies which seek to "fix." "Fixing" implies that there is something damaged, broken, or wrong with the client. There is nothing wrong with her, but she does need time and space for healing. Many current practices do not make room for this particularly important time in therapy.

Bringing our working model to bear means looking at our client as if through multiple lenses—current and past stressors and adaptation, present resources, her preferences and desires. When we understand her experience and obstacles to healing, then we consider our toolkit. Every tool is not for every problem, but a somatic focus is always appropriate because we—and our clients—are always living bodies. When we deploy our CBT or IPT or EMDR* protocols alongside somatic interventions, we support integration of body and mind so that she feels more "herself" and better prepared to mother her children.

Being-With

Somatic psychotherapists are well acquainted with "being-with." As described above, simply being in the same space provides an opportunity for our nervous system to co-regulate with the client's system. Beyond that, though, just sitting with challenging emotions, acknowledging them, and making space for them, is, in itself, an intervention, albeit a very difficult one. It is so much easier to jump to try to "fix" things than to be present to her suffering. The hardest times for clients and for therapists are when we sit together, week after week, while things do not change, and both parties begin to feel a creeping, dark hopelessness.

In fact, these may be the most important moments of the therapy. Can we sit with the client in her struggle? If we can be present to that, then we offer her something that she has never had: an environment in which she feels safe where her feelings, however unpleasant, are acceptable. The challenge for therapists is to stay with the feelings instead of disappearing from the relationship by looking for a remedy. Both of you learn to trust the process of staying with feelings, increasing her ability to tolerate the discomfort. Feeling the feelings instead of avoiding them increases emotional competency and mastery. Mastery doesn't mean control but being able to experience feelings without collapsing or being overwhelmed.

---

* Cognitive-behavioral therapy, interpersonal therapy, eye-movement desensitization and reprocessing

Connecting to the body-mind

The history of psychotherapy includes changing priorities. From the 1940s, behavioral approaches vied with psychoanalysis, ultimately giving way to cognitive therapies. At the same time, a humanistic approach emphasized relationship and allowed for the importance of emotion in treatment. But treatment approaches are not simply the conceptual darlings of theorists. They also arise from unmet needs in the population.

The formal introduction of Post Traumatic Stress Disorder (PTSD) by the American Psychiatric Association in 1980 was pivotal to the burgeoning of body-oriented therapies. When we see traumatic stress symptoms as a host of interlocking physiological and psychological experiences, somatic approaches to therapy make sense and have found support in neuroscience.

Bioenergetic psychotherapy has incorporated new findings while remaining true to underlying theory. From its psychoanalytic roots, bio takes into account the unconscious, which resides in and shows up through the body. Rather than focusing on interpretation as psychoanalysis does, bio prioritizes direct somatic experience.

Whatever school of therapy you subscribe to, you can shift toward the somatic without violating your assumptions. The body has been there in therapy all along. Somatic experience has been continually informing your thoughts and feelings, and those of your clients. You are making those connections available to awareness. In so doing, you change what is implicit to explicit.

How do you shift gears toward the somatic? Here is an exercise to explore the continuous awareness of the interplay of body experiences with mental activity. You can experience this at any moment by just taking time to check in with yourself.

Do it now. Here are the directions.

Exercise #1:   Checking In (Finding Your Own Body-Mind)

You can take the orienting position or just stay where you are. Wherever you are, notice your next breath. Just notice it.

Inhale, exhale. That's it. No judgment. No change. Just notice.

Now notice another one. Inhale, exhale. One more.

Now allow your attention to go inside your experience. What can you sense from the inside out? What is present in your belly, your chest, your throat? Do you feel the movement air makes in your body?

Can you feel the chair you sit on? The straightness or curve of your back? What do you notice in your legs and feet? How does your face feel right now?

Now notice the contents of your thoughts. Can you experience them as separate from the body sensations? Separate from each other? Are you having any thoughts that seem related to your experience, such as "my chest feels tight?" Just notice whatever you are currently experiencing with friendliness and nonjudgment.

Now let it go.

Take a moment to reflect. What was that like? What did you notice? Was there anything unexpected? How do you feel in this moment?

Make a note about your experience. Notice what happens as you write. Does this change your experience?

When checking inside, you were aware of your body experience and the thoughts that were flowing along with them. You might have had other thoughts too, seemingly unrelated ones or about the process itself. This is what I mean about being aware of the interplay of body experience with mental activity.

Somatic psychotherapies are not new, even if the approach might be new to you. The various approaches have developed many direct, clear, and effective interventions for use with your perinatal clients.

Reproductive issues are about the body, reflecting a person's sexual and parental identity

Your client may come because of fertility, pregnancy, or postpartum problems. She's emotionally overwhelmed and her sleep, nutrition, exercise/movement, and reactivity are all out of whack. No wonder she has distorted thoughts. Problem thinking occurs in people whose bodies are struggling.

Many people unrealistically believe that they can control their thoughts. Adjunctively, they believe if they could only understand their thoughts, they would be fine. There is often an unstated belief that if they were really good enough persons (good enough mothers) they would understand and thus be in control. These beliefs often accompany profound body dysregulation. When therapy focuses on helping the body to become more regulated, thinking tends to fall into line. Then clients can think rationally again and cognitive methods can be effective.

We're not just talking about good health habits. Unfortunately, there are public advocates for concrete changes in behavior, such as eating regularly, walking outside, and encouraging gratitude as a cure for mental illness. While those things can change how people feel, think, and cope, they don't cure. They are helpful but not sufficient. When I suggest therapy starting with the body, I mean as a focus for therapeutic intervention.

A person's sense of self as a sexual being derives in part from how she experiences herself from the inside out. Fertility problems will affect her thinking about her bodily self. Women who struggle to get pregnant or stay pregnant may experience their bodies as damaged, incapable, or bad. Fertility issues often strike people who have not had serious illness or injury before and can result in feeling like the body has failed in some major way. This often translates into people thinking they have failed.

Any trauma background can be reactivated by perinatal distress. Trauma fundamentally changes a woman's relationship to her body. This is due, in part, to the nature of traumatizing events. By definition, they are events in which her survival is at risk. Accidents, weather events, or being a victim of a crime can be traumatizing.

Normal childbirth, which is to say childbirth that is not experienced as traumatizing by the birthing person, is an intense experience of body, mind, and spirit. Typical experiences of childbirth generally need to be processed somatically, cognitively, and emotionally to become part of a woman's reproductive identity.

Adverse Childhood Events (ACES)

Traumatizing events are shockingly common; 12% of the US population has experienced a number of adverse childhood events sufficient to affect their health and longevity (Felitti 1993; Boyce et al. 2012). These are consequential to physical and mental health and even longevity. Childhood stress has lifetime consequences, yet we pay very little attention to mitigating the sources, such as poverty.

Birth processing happens spontaneously in most cases: women tell and retell their birth stories, sorting and organizing their experiences. However, the extreme intensity of experience in PMADs means women may need guidance through this normative process. It is safest and most respectful to assume anyone has sensitivities around the birth experience. This is the crux of a trauma-friendly stance.

A woman who has earlier trauma may find the typical somatic and emotional intensity of pregnancy, childbirth, and infant care to be particularly challenging. Even without previous trauma, childbirth is sometimes traumatic. The birthing body experiences loss, intrusion, panic during procedures, or distress due to unexpected changes, often accompanied by helplessness and terror. These experiences may become "stuck" in a woman's inner space. She may have overt re-experiencing and even develop sufficient symptoms to qualify for a diagnosis of PTSD.

Somatic interventions are experiential and efficient

Somatic interventions are experiential. Do them in the session with the client, guiding and supporting, then debriefing. Through exploration, the client has an immediate and direct experience of something new in the body. Doing the intervention with her, rather than talking about it, shows you value the bodywork. When she experiences herself differently with you, she takes away a somatic memory, a moment full of sensation, feeling, and thoughts that becomes a resource. After having the experience and putting her words to it, she is more likely to practice at home.

Intervening this way has many advantages. First, she gives you feedback immediately on her experience. You provide structure and support her as she tries something new. You mirror, attune, and reflect. You show her that her tiniest experience is important to you, so she can start to offer compassion and friendly curiosity to herself. When you attune to her inner experience, she feels heard and felt. Because she trusts you, and you think she's okay, she can start to trust herself.

Somatic interventions are quick and require only close attention to focus and report on body sensations.

Here is an example. A typical answer to the "how are you feeling?" opener might be "terrible." When you ask what feels terrible, she'll tell you she's thinking that she is a bad mother, a bad person, or that she is harming her baby because she feels so bad. Clearly, her "terrible" feeling is related to her thoughts. Redirect to sensations: where do you notice that in your body?

Using sensations instead of "feelings" is more fine-grained and less emotionally loaded. Staying with sensation keeps you out of storytelling. Attending to the sensations in the body allows her to sidestep those harsh internal judgments. Anyone could be feeling tightness in the chest, queasiness in the belly, and aching in the lower back. Those sensations don't reflect the "kind of person" or the "kind of mother" she is. They are just body sensations.

You know, of course, that those body sensations often accompany negative self-talk, frightening images, and punitive judgments about the self, but the sensations themselves are less emotionally loaded. Taking a moment to attend to body sensations gives a person a break from the incessant barrage of negative self-talk and self-images. Attending to sensation creates a simultaneous sense of distance from thought and connection to a deeper somatic self.

❧ CHAPTER 2 ❧

Body Psychotherapy for Perinatal Clients

Somatic therapies include a number of labels but have a common core. Because I am a bioenergetic therapist and trainer, I'll necessarily be using the language of bioenergetics, but the assumptions and principles apply across styles. There are three basic assumptions for a body psychotherapy approach, which I'll discuss below.

- Mind and body are a unity.
- Energy in the body is a real thing.
- Present experience is a function of past body experiences.

Mind and body are a unity

Mind and body are one thing, even though we talk about them and behave as if they are separate. Much of our childhood socialization is around denying the body and getting the mind to override the signals of the body. Specifically, we learn to wait to eat, to defecate, and for our turn to play with the truck. We must learn to sit when our bodies would prefer to run around. We must learn to hold back our tears when they're unwelcome. Over time, we teach ourselves to work through fatigue, to look happy when we are broken-hearted and to repress our feelings. We push through pain. We work hard to make a separation between our bodies and our minds, as if our minds are our "real selves" and our bodies just carriers.

Beyond this, we live our lives under pressure: financial pressure, time pressure, and social pressure. The body interprets these pressures as life-threatening. No matter how we try, our minds cannot rationalize away a body-based fear concerning our survival. We live in a state of chronic stress and distress that has become so commonplace that we do not even notice it as stressful until there is an opportunity for quiet, relaxation, or peacefulness. When those opportunities arise, we might notice how different it is to settle and soften our bodies. Or we might become anxious or overwhelmed, or we might discover that even given the opportunity, we cannot deeply relax. Who we are in our bodies constructs how we are in the world, at least in part.

Our body experiences give rise to our narrative selves, the stories we tell ourselves about our lives. A chronically stressed, tired, and over-whelmed mother is going to have a different story about her place in her family than a mother who is relaxed and comfortable in her body.

There is more about how our bodies dictate our stories in Chapter 3.

Energy is a real thing

Energy is needed for every function of our bodies, from maintaining cell health to moving us through exercise class to thinking about work. Energy in the body comes from food, oxygen, and light and can be experienced as high or low, free-flowing, or blocked. The energy we use is a manifestation of our physiology, not some esoteric flow. Because energy flows through body tissues, including liquid such as lymph, it can get blocked or stuck by muscular tension or rigidity in the con-nective tissues. When we chronically block the flow by tightening the muscles, we have chronic tension in the body.

Thinking processes are energetic processes too. The artificial separation of body and mind has led us to conceptualize thinking as something that is matter-less and energy-less. Not true! Thinking is a process that includes neural transmission but also likely includes other parts of the body. We effortlessly access memory and the parts of our brain that predict the future as we are thinking, and while thinking, we are using energy.

If you are unsure whether there are energy processes in thinking, imagine trying to do a complex problem-solving task when your blood sugar is low. Thinking requires energy. Energy in the body is neither an esoteric flow nor a metaphor. Bodies need fuel and oxygen to generate energy to live, grow, move, think, emote, and lactate.

Present experience is a function of the past

Since our bodies are affected by our histories, and our behavior and thinking are influenced by our bodies, our histories cannot help but influence our present-day beliefs and functioning. Our bodies have our history written on them and in them. I have a scar on a finger where I slammed it in a car door when I was sixteen. I have stretch marks from pregnancy, episiotomy scars, and an empty place where my tonsils used to be. Beyond any personal litany of scars and marks, we have chronic muscle tensions that occur because of behavioral patterns. This includes daily life patterns and also how we learned to manage our feelings.

Imagine you are a small child playing in the water of a fountain. You splash and look, and water sprinkles all over. You giggle and splash some more, feeling the pleasurable sensations of water and coolness and sunshine, with your feet on the ground. Allow yourself to feel immersed in the pleasure of playing in the water, feeling it, watching it, hearing it. Now imagine someone comes up and yells at you for getting wet. Assume the body posture that you might take under these circumstances: do it right now while you are reading. Notice what is happening in your body as you make this sudden shift from pleasure and play to reacting to someone yelling at you.

The way your body behaves during this imagined experience may tell you something about your patterns of responding to sudden, distressing changes. You might put up your hands as if to ward off a blow; you might twist your body away from the source of the upset; you might feel an upwelling of anger and find yourself making fists. However you responded, you likely cut off the free-flowing energy of pleasure and play. The good feelings stopped, blocked by fear, shame or anger.

If this situation occurred in an ideal world, the child would be supported by a parent and the feelings acknowledged, releasing the blocked energy. The child could then return to play.

Everyone doesn't grow up in an ideal world. Some children must stay tightly constricted to be safe, if their big feelings might get them unwanted attention. Some must tamp down feelings in order to stay connected to parents who might not be able to tolerate anger or fear or even joy. When a child grows up in this kind of environment, the body develops chronic holding. That is, the body tightens to keep the energy small and the feelings quiet. Over time, this tightness becomes chronic, so much so that it doesn't even feel like holding anymore. It just feels "normal."

However, chronic body tensions can result in distortion or even repression of our feelings. Constriction works to keep us safe, so we learn to live like that. It becomes normal, a part of us. Only later do we discover how constriction has limited us, when our characteristic patterns no longer serve us.

For example, some women don't feel anger. They might be mildly irritated or frustrated, but they don't ever feel angry. Anger isn't a "safe" or socially acceptable feeling for women to express, so they often learn how to keep it hidden. Over time, they even repress the feeling of anger in the body. Even with clearly visible signs of angry arousal, they will deny the feeling of anger. This is the product of many years of conscious and unconscious practice in keeping this feeling at bay.

Most unfortunately, chronic tensions in the body decrease energy flow in general, so other feelings also become less available. It might be socially acceptable to feel less anger, but it is a terrible shame to miss out on feeling joy, pleasure, and euphoria because the body has shut everything down.

These somatic holding patterns coincide with patterns of thinking and behavior. Body psychotherapy explores it all: chronic tensions as well as behavior and thinking are all possible entry points into the client's experience. Often, starting with direct somatic experience gives people access to themselves in a fresh, new way.

Our social interactions are intimately connected to our somatic selves, with a cumulative effect from infancy. Imagine a child who is seen as "cute." Others seek him out and engage with smiles and encouragement, which he reciprocates. Conversely, imagine an unattractive child whose social world reflects the bother of caring for her, the irritation of her presence, the stress she creates. Her social skills may develop around hiding rather than going out. In each case, the somatic self shapes social experience. We might also surmise that a deeply loved child becomes attractive as they expand into their social world. Causation flows in both directions.

When we have constricted our bodies to hold in our unacceptable feelings, our bodies change. If we make ourselves small, we may have constricted our chests and abdomens so that it is hard to breathe deeply. We may not develop the stamina and strength that living requires, so we are often fatigued. As adults, we learn to push through fatigue, once again ignoring body signals.

If our childhood experiences left us with chronic constriction in our necks and shoulders, it will be harder for us to reach out, to lift, or to stop encroachment. We might have repeated experiences of trouble with setting boundaries, or getting the love we want, or being able to "carry our weight."

The fact that our bodies carry our histories and that our behavior patterns are related to body structure does not mean that we are bound to any predetermined future or predetermined experience. It does mean, though, that our experiences can help teach us how we tend to function and recognize the patterns we've carried into the present. Then we have the flexibility to consider whether continuing those patterns serves us. Bioenergetic psychotherapy helps us to identify patterns. Moreover, it offers hope for change.

Case Example #1: Julie struggles with a challenging toddler

Julie, mother of a toddler and a six-month-old, reports feeling guilty and sad because she yelled at her toddler.

"Tell me a little about that. Can you give an example?"

As she describes a situation, I am closely watching how she holds her body, what happens to her breathing and skin color, what she does with her hands, and her eye contact as she talks. I gently ask her what she notices in her body as she tells me about this.

She looks surprised. "In my body?"

"Just see what you notice," I encourage. "You can't do this wrong."

She places a hand over her abdomen and says, "I feel a little sick right here," looking at me.

I nod, encouragingly.

"I can't believe I screamed at him. What kind of mother does that?" She looks again at me, eyes judgmental.

"So your stomach feels a little sick," I say, mirroring* her hand by touching my own abdomen. Here is a therapy choice point. Rather than addressing her self-judgment, I choose to stay with her immediate experience. "What else do you notice?"

She turns her attention back inward. "Really heavy, like I couldn't get up if I tried."

"Oohh," I say, using my voice to reflect heaviness. This is affect attunement*.

"Yeah, like no matter what, I am just going to screw up." She suddenly looks very sad.

"Mmmm," I say, reflectively. "Where do you notice that in your body?"

We are making the connection between body sensations and thinking.

She checks again. "Kind of in my shoulders."

I notice she has collapsed into her chest, barely breathing. I offer validation and watch. "It's a lot, taking care of a baby and toddler, and keeping the home fires burning, and trying to take care of yourself, too, when you are not feeling good."

"Yeah, it is a lot," she says. "It feels like a lot most days." She sinks deeper into the couch.

"I wonder if we could stand up and explore a couple of things?" I invite.

She drags herself off the couch to standing, hip tilted.

I stand too, but on both feet, facing her. I am in alignment with her, but not mirroring her stance. I'm watching, making encouraging eye contact. Her weight is mostly on the left, so that her hips are cocked left, putting a twist in her lower back. Her shoulders also stay forward and down. Her head hangs a bit. Without taking her position, I imagine what it feels like to be standing that way.

I invite her to notice what's present now that she is standing. "What is different in your body now? Anything?"

She takes stock, spontaneously shifting her weight onto both feet and straightening her spine. Note that there were no words exchanged about her posture. "Not quite as heavy," she says with mild interest.

"That sounds like a good thing," I comment. "Is that an improvement for you?"

"Yeah, a little bit," she agrees. She is still inward focused, so

---

*Mirroring and affect attunement are "mothering" skills that therapists use while developing connection and rapport. They also support the development of a body resonance that helps us have an "intuitive" sense of the client experience.

I give her space to notice whatever she's attending to. When she looks back up at me, I offer grounding as a next step.

"Would you be open to doing a little work with your feet, just to see what it is like?" Generally, people will agree to an encouraging invitation even if they are highly skeptical, especially if they have already felt a shift.

Together, we each very slowly roll a foot over a six-inch long wooden dowel, massaging deeply into toes, ball of the foot, arch, and heel. I remind her to slow down, notice the experience, and that it's okay to control the intensity of the sensation, pointing out that we want to feel the foot, not hurt it. We spend a full minute on one foot, then I ask her to put both feet on the floor and notice what she got from that exercise.

"I can feel this foot more." She indicates the one she's been working on. "It seems closer to the floor. Yeah. I can feel the other leg more, though," she adds with a giggle.

I nod, smile, and suggest working on the other foot.

After she has worked with both feet, I ask her to check in again with her whole body. "Not so bad," she admits. "I feel a little lighter."

"Mmhmm, lighter," I say. "Do you remember what we were talking about before?"

"Oh, yes," she says, face dimming a bit. "My little guys. Yeah, some days are hard." This is a much softer and more realistic formulation than "I am a bad mother." She is developing a bit of compassion for herself as her body feels lighter.

I invite her to share what she's thinking now that she's more in touch with her body. "Do you want to say any more about that?"

As she begins to talk, I watch her posture carefully; when I see her shoulders starting to collapse and her chest to become concave, I straighten my back and take a deep breath. Without apparently noticing it, she mirrors my shifting body attitude, and I listen carefully to what she has to say about her children and her shame and distress. Her body wants to assume a posture of shame and hopelessness; she is counteracting this by standing up on both feet and by maintaining a straight back. This is happening without overt coaching but by simply inviting her to attend to what is going on in her body while she is talking about her children and how she feels. I note with her that she feels different about the whole topic from a position of standing up on both feet than she does collapsed onto the couch.

This brief example gives a bit of the flavor of the body-specific aspects of this type of psychotherapy. Future chapters offer specific techniques.

❧ CHAPTER 3 ❧

Body-Mind Basics

Links between body and mind

Our experiences occur in time, and they take up time. They are real, concrete events that our bodies live through. Our bodies have experiences and then our minds explain the experiences. In a way, our minds tell us stories to make those experiences coherent. Sometimes those narratives are realistic and supportive. Sometimes our narratives are distorted, unrealistic, and even splintered.

We can explore our stories by talking about them, and we can reshape them by having new and different body experiences. Different experiences generate a spontaneous reorganization of our internal, often unconscious, narratives. Because they are omnipresent, we assume they are the truth. These "core beliefs" are assumed to be the truth of the world, but instead they are representations of body experience. Recent developments in our understanding of the autonomic nervous system (ANS) have shed some light on this process. (Deb Dana has been working with the narrative/ANS interplay in therapy for some time now. See Dana 2018.)

We all have stories about our lives. This includes the Big Stories about how we got to be the way we are and the little ones, like annoying traffic during school drop-off. We experience something and we tell ourselves and others about our experience. This is how we make sense of our world.

Clients explore their stories by talking with us. Stories change when people change, when new information arises, or there is a new experience. Novel somatic experiences generate a spontaneous reorganization of our internal narratives.

Stories of danger, connection, and survival all arise from activation of our ANS. Actually, every experience in a body arises there; without continuous ANS functioning we couldn't survive. ANS runs the body chemically, electrically, on the level of organ function, and also in its responsiveness to the environment.

Stephen Porges's polyvagal theory of the ANS (2011) has provided us with some new ways to conceptualize body-mind integration. The great gift of the polyvagal theory to psychotherapists lies in the "poly" part. Porges has shown how the different parts of the vagus nerve have various functions within the parasympathetic nervous system (PNS).

You may have learned about the ANS as a dual system, in which the sympathetic part gets activated when there is danger, inciting an organism to "fight or flight or freeze," and the PNS deactivates that part when danger is over. The PNS calms the system after the sympathetic activates it.

It turns out that this tidy model is incomplete. Instead, the PNS has multiple branches.

Sympathetic and PNS are activated simultaneously. They function coherently to keep you alive, active, and connected.

Beyond that, our ANS informs our thinking processes and provides the raw data for those narratives we construct. The ventral vagal nerve of the PNS enervates the head, face, upper chest, and diaphragm. This part is the executive level—in charge when everything is going along just fine. It manages our energy and our connection to the world and other people. The sound of a voice, a soft touch on the face or lips, or the sight of a smiling face stimulate the ventral vagus. When these stimuli fall within a "safe" range, the vagal activation and sense of well-being increases. Porges refers to the ventral vagal as the "social engagement system," the top of the hierarchy that includes sympathetic and dorsal vagal branches. When the social engagement part is in charge, we feel good; we are capable of learning new things and we can connect to other people.

Danger stimulates the sympathetic branch to dominate, activating the body for action. The body changes (pupils widen, respiration accelerates, heart rate goes up, adrenaline flows, digestion slows, capillaries expand) to prepare you to fight, run away, freeze in hypervigilance, or save your child from traffic.

The third part of the "polyvagal" system is the dorsal vagal, which enervates from below the diaphragm down the back. Dorsal vagal activation is involved in "rest and digest" and the slowing, numbing, and immobility that can happen when we are feeling overwhelmed.

When sympathetic activation gets high quickly, the dorsal vagal exerts the "vagal brake" on the heart, capping the level to which heart rate can increase. The next step is dorsal vagal activation to slow movement, thinking, and narrowing the field of perception. When our dorsal vagal system is overactive, we experience affect flattening, numbing of sensation, and excessive sleepiness.

The mind makes stories to go with these body experiences. This is one of the most important things to remember. The mind makes stories to go with the experiences generated by the ANS, all the time. This is the source of our stories. Even if we learned things from family members, they have become our stories through our own ANS interaction with them.

The construction of narrative around ANS experience is clearly apparent in trauma, where the distorted beliefs arise out of either sympathetic hyperarousal or dorsal vagal hypoarousal. The world is unsafe (because I feel threatened). Or the world is too much (because I cannot tolerate the stimulation and my ANS is in retreat).

Long-standing patterns of ANS arousal influence our stories about relating. When everything is going well, you feel safe and connected. The ventral vagal branch of your PNS, where the social engagement system resides (the top-level branch of the ANS), is in charge.

The neuroception (pre-perception sensing) of danger sends the ANS systems into alert mode. Think about that: neuroception precedes perception. It is hard to conceptualize but we have all experienced it. If there is a slither in the leaves near your feet, you'll find your heart racing and your breathing affected before your thinking mind registers the event. If a ball whizzes past your head, you'll duck before you even perceive that the ball is there.

Deb Dana (2018) suggests that our ANS interprets the world, and our minds make a story to match. Imagine you are walking down the street and have a neuroception of danger as a person walks toward you. Your brain starts pattern matching visually ("Who does that look like? Oh, is it him?") and emotionally ("When have I felt like this before?"). A story arises. Those stories then guide your behavior and your overall emotional responses.

Our ANS is the world to us. We act as if the world is out there, existing independently of our perceptions, but we cannot experience it directly. Our sensory organs and nervous system filter the world. This physiological fact means our personal reality cannot reflect an "objective" reality, if such a thing exists. We operate from the perspective of our body, influenced by prior experience. The world is safe or dangerous, full of challenges and stimulation or dull and colorless. Our stories reflect our experience.

Therapy gives people a novel experience which can lead to changes in their lives. From a somatic perspective, change at the body level can stimulate change at the cognitive level.

Thinking, emotions, behavior

Our real-life experiences involve the continuous flow of thoughts, emotions, and activity and their intersection in our somatic life. The flow contains these different aspects, which we can look at separately.

Thinking is the often-semiconscious set of processes that our minds engage in: it includes remembering, fantasizing about the future, analyzing, and generating new ideas. It is often automatic and includes internal verbalizations (the things we say to ourselves) or internal images—whether visual or sensory—passing quickly or slowly. Thinking, as we've seen above, is a result of somatic experience. One therapeutic goal is to help clients become more conscious of their thinking.

Our emotion categories are happy, sad, angry, afraid, disgusted, or ashamed. Emotions are culturally defined and prescribed, such that people from different cultures experience culture-specific emotions. The clarity of our feeling is affected by the label we give it. Emotions or feelings are distinctly a body experience with a mental label. "Having a feeling" means a lot of things, including intuition, memory, or describing a felt sense.

Contemporary neuroscience models (Barrett & Russell 2014) suggest that emotion is not universal but culturally and individually created in the moment. Our brains are perpetually making predictions about what will happen next, both in the world and in our bodies. Our predictions include labeling our feelings.

Verbal labels make a difference to the kind of experience you have. Calling an experience a "challenge" vs. calling it a "stress" will ease the stress in the body. Labeling a specific type of anger means that you'll feel differences within the anger, rather than a whole flood of incomprehensible affects. We can encourage clients to create personal labels that go beyond traditional categories by asking "what do you notice?" or "what is that like?" When clients can describe their personal varieties of emotion, the feelings become tolerable. This fine analysis is called "emotional granularity."

Special cases: Guilt, regret, disappointment, failure

Some feelings focus more on thinking than sensation. Guilt is an excellent example. A client who reports feeling "guilty" will have trouble locating that feeling in the body but might locate shame or

---

Emotion

Emotion is movement in the body that has a verbal/cognitive label attached. As therapists, we can help people to develop their emotional granularity, or the ability to parse out different varieties of emotion. Ask your client to notice what is happening in her body while she is experiencing something.

Anything counts. This exercise is likely very new and fresh for a client. You want to support her experience of turning toward her body sensations.

A woman might notice that her eyes are watering and that her throat feels tight. That may feel like sadness to her, but don't jump to a label. I might ask what else she can notice? Any sensations in the chest, for example? When I hear tight throat and wet eyes, it may or may not be sadness, but it most certainly is the effort of holding back some sort of emotional expression. If she wasn't trying so hard NOT to feel something, what might she feel? She is trying to stop the movement of the body that is feeling or emotion.

---

sadness. Her story might be a tale of falling short, and she feels "bad" when she thinks her children are being shortchanged by having her as a mother. No wonder she's constricted, tense, pulled in, or flattened by those thoughts. Some people become so tense while pondering their own badness they become numb to body sensations.

Regret and disappointment attach thoughts to sensations associated with sadness and anger. Finding the emotion under the thought requires attention to the body, rather than the narrative. For some people, accessing the body is hard because the storyline is so loud.

When the thinking is more available than the body sensations, we therapists have two places to work. We can begin with the thoughts and ask her to monitor changes in her experiences of her body as we go. As the body changes, the sensations become more accessible. Alternatively, we can work directly with the body by focusing on sensations, thereby skipping the negative self-judgment.

A note about rage and raging

Postpartum rage is such a common and terrifying complaint, it even has its own hashtag. Rage is a feeling, and raging is a behavior, a critical distinction.

Rage is a strong, intense feeling, not anger but akin. Raging is the behavior of explosive discharge of rage with an intent to hurt. Rage feels huge in the body, and in fact, the rageful body is often quite large as a person will spread their arms, take a wide stance with their feet, extend the spine to its fullest length, and make the eyes and mouth very large, even showing teeth. In raging, there is fast movement, as if from pent-up energy, which comes out through gestures, screaming or shouting, and possibly foot stamping, running, or striking out.

Rage, when expressed toward a person, is where the problem arises. Anger, suppressed over time without acknowledgment or any chance to discharge the energy of it, can accumulate into rage. Alternatively, rage can be a response to severe deprivation that occurred at any time in the person's life. Postpartum rage that arises out of needs unmet in one's own childhood sometimes shows up without apparent cause.

The feeling is not a problem. It is a feeling. It can be hard to tolerate and may generate a lot of problem thinking, but the feeling is just a feeling, albeit a big, scary one.

Raging, which is the explosive, hurtful discharge of rage, is damaging to both the recipient and the mother who is rageful. The behavior is the problem. Not the feeling.

Poor mother: Even before she's discharged the rage, she's full of shame and guilt. She may be unable to apologize because she is so ashamed and overwhelmed. Instead of making amends, she exacerbates the situation, because admitting both what she did and that she feels bad about it, at that very moment, is impossible. Her shame is so enormous that the only thing to do is pretend that everything is either okay or that the child is to blame. This is the pattern that results in families "never talking about" difficult things, thus losing opportunities to strengthen relationships through repairing the rupture.

Shark music cues rage

Nobody had a perfect childhood; nobody had perfect parents. Every one of us had places where our emotional needs were not met or where we were met with something frightening. Because those memories are still tucked away in the part of our brain called "implicit memory," we can be activated into feeling dread even if there is nothing scary in the present. This triggered dread is so overwhelming that it can result in rage.

Parenting infants and young children is hard work. It's physically and emotionally demanding, often continuously. Some parts will feel harder than others. We may feel a sense of ominous foreboding at times. Some parenting programs refer to this feeling as a response to our "shark music" (see Powell et al. 2013), a play on the feeling of foreboding activated by the ominous music from the old movie *Jaws*. Shark music alerts our ANS to danger.

We react due to activation of frightening implicit memories from very early childhood. Because they are implicit, they are not available to consciousness, so there's no real explanation for why we suddenly feel so terrified or so rageful. We're activated into fight, flight, freeze, or collapse. Our bodies say something terrible is happening or about to happen.

Life with infants and toddlers gives us a lot of opportunity to encounter sharks, and of course shark music is individual. Some parents tolerate crying babies but can't handle preschool defiance. Some are cool with chaos but panic with vomit or illness. One mother reported that she couldn't stand it when her two girls fought. She needed to leave or scream. She later recalled her mother terrifyingly brandishing a wooden spoon during a sibling squabble. Her mother's shark music also may have been kids fighting.

Because the sense of dread or anger isn't connected to an explicit memory, the shark music feels like a prediction, as if something terrible is going to happen. The mother feels a huge surge of emotion—anger, say, or terror—and feels like she must stop it at any cost, even if it means screaming at her child. The implicit memory is detached from its roots, so she can't tell it is just a memory generating a feeling. Feelings cannot predict the future.

In this case, unfortunately, something terrible does happen. Because of the intolerable feeling, she screams at the child. She reacts in an extreme, historical way to a here-and-now situation, because she's being haunted by memories. Being screamed at by her mother is the terrible thing that her body feared. Now, though, she is the mother.

The fear she feels is of a long-ago shark, but it puts her in the position of creating those fears in her children. Without an understanding of how implicit memories can activate present-day reactions, parents and children are stuck in the threads of early developmental trauma that travels through generations, even in the absence of explicit memories.

When parents grasp the nature of implicit memories, they have a label of "shark music" to pause and reflect. When they are feeling a flood of distressing emotion, asking, "Am I hearing shark music?" allows a more compassionate self-gaze. That moment can make all the difference.

When shark music is activated, a mother may be going through a cascade of frightening or confusing thoughts and feelings. Her thoughts about the baby are important, as they can render a lot of information.

Case Example #2: Nicole's shark music

When her infant cried and was hard to console, Nicole often thought that the baby boy was mad at her, and deep inside she wondered if he could see her thoughts. She wondered what he knew about her, if he knew that she was struggling to feel connected. She even wondered if he thought she was a bad mother or a bad person.

Nicole had trouble articulating these thoughts. It is easy to be dismissive of ideas that are so clearly irrational, and Nicole struggled to even allow herself to know what she is thinking. She was also afraid that anyone who knew what she was thinking would hear her thoughts as crazy.

Worse, she was afraid to even talk about them in therapy, because of the danger that I might confirm her worst fears. Her sense of inadequacy increased every time the baby cried. Her baby cried a lot, partly because she was so agitated and fearful in her body that she was tentative in how she touched and held him. She could feel his judgment as he looked at her, and while she knew intellectually that he was unable to judge her, she felt overwhelmed and inadequate and wanted to run away. It took some time for her to share these experiences in therapy.

The concept of shark music took away a lot of the self-judgment and self-blame. I asked her to pay attention to how her insides felt when the baby cried. She had no trouble describing it and was even able to generate a facsimile in the office without the baby. Her stomach was upset, her chest tight, her heart racing and there was a very clear idea that something terrible was going to happen immediately. When she could allow herself to notice her thinking, she realized she was imagining some faceless social worker kicking in the door and taking her baby away.

We did some grounding and breathing to settle her sympathetic nervous system, and she checked in again. Her belly was quieter, and she could take a fuller breath.

Pressing her feet into the floor, she makes up a mantra: "There are no sharks here." With a giggle, she says, "Now I'm imagining that social worker as a shark, swimming far out to sea." She sobers. "But I still wonder if my baby thinks I'm a bad mom, the way he looks at me."

"How does it feel?" I ask.

By now she's figured out I mean in her body, so she tunes inward. "Yeah, tight. A little sick. But I know a little baby's not really sitting there wishing he had a different mother. Maybe I'm wishing I were a different mother."

"With a different baby? One that didn't cry so much?"

She looks shocked, then laughs. "No, he's mine and I want him. I wish he'd come with directions, though."

Nicole's shark music was loud and clear. Her baby cried a lot, and she struggled to console him. It is very likely some part of her did think he was a bad baby, because of all his crying. She may have been angry at this bad baby, much like a toddler throwing his doll on the floor for a pretend crime. She might have had some barely conscious fantasies of leaving him to cry, of running away, or handing him off to someone else.

Unconscious management of her feelings turned into a projection, a defense in which a mother attributes her unacceptable thoughts and feelings to somebody else. In Nicole's case, her baby was angry with her for being a bad mother. Not only could Nicole not accept her own feelings, she projected them onto her baby and assumed he was judging her, despite her logic that babies don't judge.

The painful tension between her emotional thinking and her rational thinking made her genuinely less capable of caring for her baby effectively. Her reactions flooded and overwhelmed her and left her unable to function.

The notion of shark music and the acknowledgment that we have weird irrational thoughts and feelings about our babies can create space for self-compassion. Self-compassion is a first step. It is hard to be compassionate toward a demanding infant when we are harsh with ourselves.

Shark music and PMADS

Nicole was too activated to respond to her child from a here-and-now adult perspective. This is just what happens when we are reacting to our inner experience of danger and fear and can't see what the child needs. This limitation means nothing about the person except that she is activated. She's not a bad person or a bad parent.

Our clients want to meet their babies' needs and often can't recognize their own. In this instance, Nicole's needs are high. Shark music tells a story about a childhood need that went unmet. As therapists, we can help parents to reflect on this, based on the body sensations of reaction.

If parents can take time to ask themselves, "What do I need right now?" they make a little space before reacting. Just noting a need helps them shift gears and step back into parenting. Adults can wait to have needs met but only if they know that someone, even if it is oneself, is paying attention to that need.

In some ways, perinatal mood and anxiety disorders are like continuous shark music. The ongoing arousal, activation, and excessive thinking can feel like being in the water with a great white shark who is ready for lunch. The danger signals are false, but the parent doesn't know it. She's stuck in believing that there really is a shark, or worse, that she is the problem. In her mind, she is a bad mother or perhaps a crazy person. Should she be afraid of sharks or afraid that she's crazy?

Either way, she's upset, overwhelmed, hiding her feelings, and wishing it would all go away.

Taming sharks is a lot of what maternal psychotherapy is about. Bioenergetic techniques help us to get to the feeling parts of the perinatal stories, and then we can help mothers write a new next chapter.

CHAPTER 4

Creating Somatically Safe Spaces

Meeting the body's needs: a foundation for effective therapy

Families are often unprepared for the emotional experience of adding a baby to the family. A baby's deep dependency can trigger a woman's own longing for closeness and connection. If she's not getting those needs met, she'll find it hard to care for her baby. While we can't control what happens in our clients' homes, we can help them think about how to meet their very real needs. Everyone needs to be well-fed, get proper rest, and have someone who is kind and interested in how they are doing. This includes the entire perinatal support team: grandparents, spouses, other children, even family friends. Babies, of course, need to be held and fed and cared for and held some more. Mothers are not the sole providers. In the early postpartum period, a mother needs much more care and kindness from others than she is likely to acknowledge.

Without support, how can she get the required nourishment, rest, and protection? The outside world is demanding on parents of newborns. The more children in the family, the more the mother needs time and space to be held and hold the new baby. Holding means not just the mother holding the baby, but the mother having the experience of being held and cared for in both concrete and emotional ways.

If you can help mothers plan their postpartum experience, focus on the body. Making babies is a physically demanding business and making milk to keep those babies growing also demands calories, fluids, and rest. We have a societal notion that pregnancy is a special time, but once the baby is born, business returns to usual. Mothers are expected to be back doing all the things that they did before the baby: family, work, community responsibilities. As a society, we are not respectful of the mother's very reasonable needs for support and, by extension, her family's.

Food, rest, kind listening, and space to be with all the new experiences of childbirth and newborn care are essentials, not luxuries, for the mother. Treating emotional distress will be more effective if we have given attention to the foundation of somatic developments in the early postpartum period.

Perinatal bodies

Perinatal women have a lot going on, somatically. For many, the experiences of pregnancy, childbirth, and newborn care present a previously unknown level of somatic connection. The continuous dance of body contact, connection, separation, and regulation between an infant and mother is obvious to the observer. Less obvious is the way the body of the perinatal client influences and is influenced by the other bodies she relates to. The continuous moment-to-moment body focus is a lot to process, and the rest of the household can also be taken by surprise.

Therapists may also be surprised by the body-ness of being with a perinatal client. Whether you realize the role of your body in the therapy, it is working for you or against you. Being oriented to the somatic interplay helps therapists use this energy well.

In all psychotherapy, the connection between client and therapist is vitally important. It is a body-level experience that neither of you may have words for. Somatic interventions slide under cognitive defenses. That is, working directly with body experiences accesses emotional states that can lead a client to feeling vulnerable, so the therapist-client relationship needs to be a better-than-average safe place. You, the therapist, become the heart and soul of emotional safety for your client. Therapists hold space for everything the client brings, including things they're not aware of. This is particularly important with perinatal clients.

Therapists need energy and focus to hold this space, to avoid zoning out or getting dysregulated when the work becomes intense, and to be both emotionally present and a watchful witness. Holding space is a skill, just as being with feelings is a skill. We must know ourselves well to hold space effectively.

Knowing our own inner space isn't a skill but a process, supported by somatic exercises. Somatic therapists of every stripe do their own somatic work. A daily practice of body awareness and expressive exercises, plus ongoing therapy and supervision, helps bioenergetic therapists prepare to be present.

Creating a safe therapy environment

We create safety even before we meet our clients. Here are some elements that support a sense of safety.

- Reliable, consistent communication. The client knows how to get in touch.
- Office space is private and contained.
- Train your online clients to make a protected space for their sessions with tissues, water, cozy blankets, and privacy.

- Protect clients from seeing others in your waiting room. Mothers coming for therapy do not want to encounter their bosses or their neighbors as they arrive or leave.
- If you have a baby-friendly practice, ensure there is a comfortable place for babies too. That means that mothers do not worry that baby noises will disturb others, that there is a pleasant place to nurse the baby, that there is a place for changing diapers.
- If you also see people who struggle with fertility issues or who have had reproductive losses, "safety" may mean a space that is not overtly baby-oriented.
- Limit stimulation in your space. Mothers are usually coming from a hugely overstimulating environment (crying babies, demanding family members, television screens, dogs barking), and finding a quiet, gentle, undemanding place in your office can feel like a vacation even before their session begins.

Overload

There are benefits of turning down the sensory stimulation. First, from a quiet, still space, people will have more awareness of stimulation in their everyday life. Second, they will have an opportunity to attend to how their bodies respond to stimulation of different kinds. Decreasing the stimulation load opens more attention to sensations and feelings within. Organizing your office to manage stimulation allows clients to experience themselves.

You can explore this for yourself. Take note of your everyday environment. Notice the stimulation: that means what you see, hear, smell, feel on your skin, and even what you "sense" in terms of the energy or vibration of a place and people. What is it like for you to "turn down the volume" on the stimulation? Turn off the music or video and notice what it feels like. If you have a lot of visual clutter, clear an area (such as a table or shelf) and notice what it is like to allow your gaze to rest on that space. Open a window to let the wind blow through and clear out any smells.

Creating "presence"

Presence is not about presentation. It's not about how you appear to your clients but about how much of yourself you can bring to the interaction. The more you are self-aware and self-possessed, the more "you" will be available in the therapy room.

We all are trained to know that the therapist-client relationship is a contributor to successful therapy. There is "something" that a good therapist has that makes her clients feel better just by being with her. Research tells us much variability in client outcomes is due to these kinds of "process variables" rather than the mode of therapy.

Somatic therapies note explicitly that the therapist herself is a critical component of care. There are specific skills involved in that elusive quality known as "presence." These skills support the overall process of becoming more completely yourself, which underlies a strong sense of presence. The exercises in the next chapter support the development of presence. They are also useful for clients.

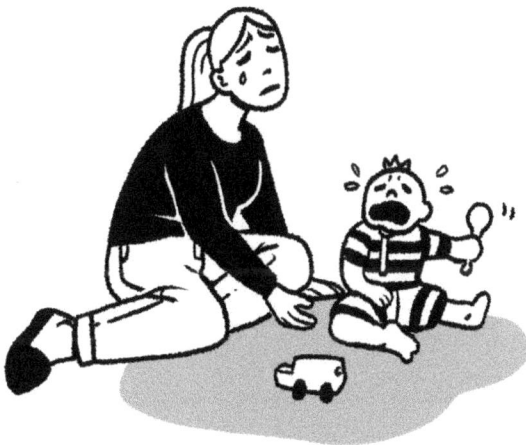

❦ CHAPTER 5 ❦

Therapist Self Skills

This chapter presents six exercises for you to use to increase your self-awareness and comfort with somatic interventions. Create some space and time for yourself to work through them. Take time before and after each one to reflect on what you notice. Use the space in this book or a journal notebook to record your reflections. Your notes will help you process your experience and will also serve as a reminder about how doing this work felt when you were new to it. That helps you understand your clients' experiences of it.

Exercise #2A: Focusing Attention

Sound

Listen for a moment, then choose a sound in your environment. Direct your attention to the sound. Stay attentive to the sound for the space of a few breaths, noticing whatever arises.

What happens as you pay more attention to the sound? Does the experience change? Does your attention want to go elsewhere? Bring your attention back to the sound and notice how it is to begin again.

Now release your attention to that particular sound.

Variation

If you have a chime or bell, try this exercise using it. Ring the bell and then just listen. Listen through the entire experience of the vibration of the bell making sound. Notice how things change and how they stay the same. When the sound has completely died away, notice if you can still hear it in your sensory memory.

Returning to everyday attention, check in with yourself. What did you get from that exercise?

Visual

Anywhere you are, notice what you see. Take in the properties of the visual field in front of you—shapes, colors, positions of objects. Feel free to look around the room. Feel yourself soaking up the images of objects you see.

Now rest your gaze on one place and allow the image of that space to come to you. Rather than seeking it out, just be present with your eyes and let the image or images arise in your awareness.

Notice if your mind wants to label and categorize. Know that you can experience without that mental activity. Rest your attention on one object in your gaze. Notice your mental activity as you do this.

When you are ready to leave that object, gently move your gaze elsewhere. Is something else calling for your attention? Can you let that object come to you?

When you are ready to stop, take a moment to shift the distance of your gaze. Look near, then far. How has your visual perception shifted?

Smell

Allow yourself to notice smells. Close your eyes if you wish and orient your attention to your sense of smell. Take time to attend to anything you can sense this way. Again, notice if your mind wants to label your experiences. Do thoughts, memories, images arise? Refocus on the smell.

Variation

You can do this activity by choosing a scent. Perhaps you'll zest a lemon and breathe in the aroma, or your morning coffee can be the stimulus. Notice how your attention is different when you have actively selected the smell. Notice what comes up, but keep returning your attention to the smell.

Skin sensations

Bring your attention to your body as a whole. Allow your awareness to rest in the envelope of your skin, that amazing organ that holds your viscera, bones, muscles, connective tissues, gases, and fluids in a resilient, receptive container. Your skin is a boundary between your inside and outside, holding and managing information from both places. Your skin is a big organ with a lot of receptors. Allow for many experiences in different parts of your skin. Notice any sensations. You may feel pressure where you are sitting, air moving across you, temperature, the texture of whatever your skin is touching. Take time. Notice how your attention deepens into awareness of subtle sensations. For example, you may notice the breath on your upper lip as you inhale and exhale. Let the experience happen.

What do you notice? Notice if labeling the experience changes it.

This exercise allows you to explore the interplay of sensation and perception, noticing how attention itself can change the experience. Before moving on, jot down some notes about what happened. Which sensory channels are most salient for you? Which did you like the best? The least? Are there thoughts, images, memories, or fantasies that relate to your experiences? Note, also, if this exercise is fatiguing. It takes energy to pay close attention.

Exercise #2B: Focused Attention on the Body

You can do this exercise from any position. If you like, you can adopt the orienting position (see Exercise #1), but it is not necessary.

Take a moment to notice the space you are in. Notice sounds, smells, the light, and shadows. Then allow your attention to move inside your body.

First, attend to your body as a whole. With compassionate curiosity, notice what sensations are present. Sensations can be anything from a tightness to shakiness to feeling expansive and loose. Observe how your mind responds to these sensations. Make space inside your attention to experience them for a few breaths. Notice if they shift as you pay attention.

Now go a bit deeper and rest your attention inside your throat. Gently attend to your throat. What is present there? What can you notice? How is it to just be with the sensations in your throat? If you like, you can rest a hand on your throat and see how that changes your experience.

Next, slide your attention to your chest, bringing the same compassionate curiosity. What is here, now? What do you notice? How does it change? A hand over your heart may make a change. Explore your experience.

When you have attended to the sensations in your chest, move your attention to your belly. Allow for the rise and fall of sensation. Notice what is present. Notice what might be hiding and offer your kind attention. Stay with the sensations in your belly to watch them arise and fall.

When you have attended to your throat, chest, and belly, allow your attention to rest again on your body as a whole. Take in your whole body, sitting, lying, or standing in space. Check to see if there are any parts calling for attention. If yes, offer them your attention in a kindly way.

As you draw this exercise to a close, make a gentle note of anything you wish to remember. When you end, intentionally say goodbye before you move your attention elsewhere. When you come back into everyday attention, take a moment to reflect on any effects of these exercises.

Exercise #3: Daily Check-In with Noting

With practice, you can learn to check in with yourself quickly. Practicing focused attention to the senses and the body, as you did in the previous exercises, prepares you for a quick regular check-in. It's a rapid assessment in which you ask yourself, "How am I doing right now?"

You'll check on body experiences, including sensations, emotions, and energy.

A check-in can be as quick as three breaths.

Plant your feet on the floor, whether you are sitting or standing. Feel your connection to the ground. Now exhale. Blow the breath out, as long as you can, then allow a spontaneous inhalation. Feel your body from the inside. You can probably feel more as you've just increased your available oxygen and expanded your torso.

As you exhale the second time, scan your inner space. What do you notice?

Inhale again and exhale. Continuing with your inner scan, is there anything that needs your attention? Make a gentle mental note. When will you attend to it? If not now, when?

That's it. This simple check-in can help you notice early indicators of tension, irritability, and stress, and expansion, pleasure, and joy. When you remember to come back to those items that you noted, you tell yourself that you matter. This is a powerful message for your somatic self. Check in with yourself regularly, multiple times a day.

How can you remind yourself to check in regularly? Some of my clients send themselves messages or set up reminders on their phones. Some people use regularly occurring external cues. Checking in helps you to address your needs before they become overwhelming.

Exercise #4: Dual Focus: Being Present to Yourself While You Are with Other People

This is an exercise in presence. Holding yourself in awareness as you hold awareness of another is a skill. Maintaining this dual awareness goes beyond empathy.

In empathy, you lean into awareness of what the other person's experience might be like. In presence, you maintain your own self-awareness while you are holding awareness of the other person. Because you are continuously influencing each other, this can be a little like juggling, but it's eminently satisfying to both therapist and client.

Now that you have experience in checking in with yourself, take that skill into your interactions. If you have a partner who will explore with you, so much the better. Otherwise, just do this exercise while you are sitting with a friend or family member, either in conversation or not. You might let them know you're doing an exploration just for everyone's comfort.

Notice yourself first. Feet connected, breathing in place, aware of whatever shows up. Make a soft note of how you are. Now allow your attention to go toward the other person.

What do you notice about the other person? Information will come to you via visual, auditory, olfactory, and interoceptive systems. That is, you'll see, hear, smell, and have a body awareness of the other person. You may have skin sensations that are related to their presence.

Notice the other person and notice what impact the other person has on your body and mind. You can try looking at them and then looking away. How do you experience that shift? If you keep the other person in mind as you look away, do you feel different?

Try looking deeply at the other person. Imagine that your eyes are taking them in, looking into all of them. If your partner is willing, you can play here with eye contact. How does eye contact affect your feeling of yourself? Can you still feel your connection to the ground and your breath?

Toggle your attention back and forth, so you check on yourself and then check on how you experience the other person. See how it is to keep this awareness of self and other through conversation and activities.

Explore keeping your self-awareness intact while interacting in other relationships. What do you notice?

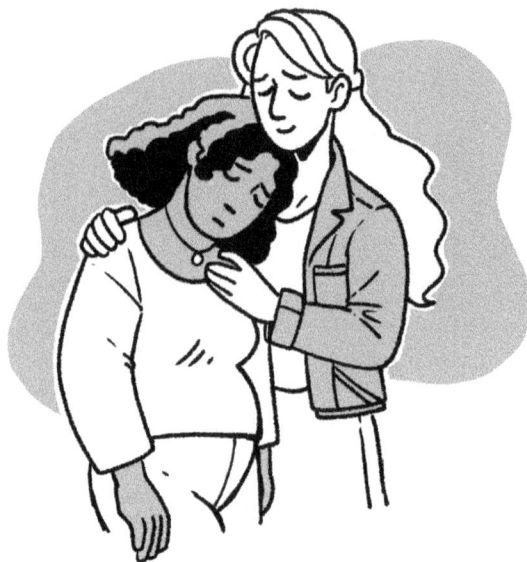

Bringing your full presence to therapy can be hard, especially with challenging cases, or when your life is intruding on your thoughts. Sometimes you need to clear your own space before you can step into presence.

You can "tidy your space" by using a focusing activity. Focusing, discovered by Eugene Gendlin, teaches you to notice the "felt sense" of the body that isn't exactly an emotion or a basic sensation. Instead, it is a "sense" that you experience at the body level that has some meaning for you.

Exercise #5:   Clearing Space

Choose a position that allows you to feel into your torso. Your back will be fairly straight and your chest open, so breath moves easily. You can sit, stand, or lie down.

To clear your space, take time to be with yourself for a moment and check in. Notice anything in your throat, chest, or belly. Allow yourself to tune into those parts of your body. Don't worry if you don't notice anything.

Now ask yourself this question. "Is there anything in the way of me being all okay?"

Take some time to let that question resonate in your body, no matter if your mind wants to override it. Just wait and notice if anything shows up in your body. You don't have to label whatever comes up. Just acknowledge it. It can just be "something." Maybe you notice "something" in your belly. There's a sensation, a feeling, a felt sense. Something that arose when you asked what was getting in the way of being all okay.

When you notice it, give it friendly, kind attention and let it unfold as it will. You can gently check to see what it might be about. Maybe it's a worry you have about finances. Just label that, gather up all the parts, including any trailing threads, and put it away on a shelf. Don't get caught in the details. Just imagine carefully putting everything connected to that felt sense away.

Don't worry that you'll never find it again. It'll be there when you want to consider it, but for right now it is safely put away. Now bring your attention back to your whole self. Resting again in awareness, ask yourself again, "Is there anything in the way of me being all okay?"

Wait.

Either you're all okay or you're not, and if you're not, a felt sense will arise. Treat it just like the last one, with kind regard, and gently tidy it onto a shelf. Continue in the same way until the space feels clear. If things try to escape the shelf, gently return them. There is no need to be harsh or to judge yourself or the felt sense. You are tidying up the inner space for now.

When the space is clear, do a full check-in. Notice your breath. Notice how your body sinks into the surfaces it touches. Sense the openness inside. Once you have cleared the space, you are ready to be present to whatever arises in your life or in your therapy practice.

Tracking energy and arousal

Somatic psychotherapists are aware of a client's body state, tracking changes in energy, attention, and arousal. We pay attention at this level because we help clients to stay within a zone of tolerance for the processing they are doing in session. We have learned to watch and listen for changes in the ANS of our clients. As usual we learn this best by practicing on ourselves.

Exercise #6: Observing Your Own Energetic Flow

Get a full-length mirror and observe your skin and your musculature.

Many people automatically move to self-judgment when looking in the mirror. If you find yourself thinking negative thoughts about your body's appearance, set them aside. Imagine you are a scientist, observing energy in the human body. At the moment, this body happens to be you. Bring your attitude of compassionate curiosity to this exercise.

Wearing shorts and a tank top will help, as you will be able to see your body more completely. While looking, try for a dual focus. Notice what you observe in the mirror while checking inward on your experience. What is it like to see your body and feel yourself at the same time?

Let yourself have time to settle into the task. Slow your breathing and bring a soft, noncritical gaze to the mirror. Look! There you are.

- First, just observe your skin. Note the colors and textures of your skin across different parts of your body. Do things change as you watch? Just notice.
- Now look for visible tension or relaxation. Where are your shoulders sitting? Is your weight balanced on your two feet? How does your internal experience of tension/relaxation match up with what you are seeing?

- Does your breathing generate movement in your body? What do you see and, at the same time, what do you feel?
- Using your soft gaze, be aware of any impressions, even if you aren't sure what they mean or if they're "real." You're working in a new area here. Be open to what you notice, even if it's different from what you expect.

When you feel you've taken in as much as you can, change your body state by engaging in vigorous movement, such as shaking all over, for a couple of minutes.

- Shake for two minutes by the clock. That can feel like a long time.
- Stop shaking. Notice what it is like to stop moving. Notice the feeling of movement left over in your body. Using your soft gaze, observe again.
- You likely can easily see changes in your skin color. What else do you notice? How does your visual observation track with what you feel inside?
- Watch your skin as the internal agitation of shaking subsides. What do you notice now? Think about how you felt at the very beginning of the exercise. How does your present state compare to this?

From this more settled place, try activating your legs by stomping your feet or kicking hard at a pillow on the floor. The largest muscles of your body are in your legs, and activation that starts here will move up. Activate, then take time to notice changes in your body appearance. Feel the energy in your legs while you watch the skin and muscles in your mirror. What happens to your face while these changes are going on in your body? When you feel heat, does your face change color? As the heat cools, are there visible changes?

Stay with it, watching, noticing, holding it all in your awareness. Notice the sensations associated with the body settling. Notice your breathing, body tensions, color. How do these compare to the very first look you took?

Now consider this: Can you influence the energy in your body by what you are thinking? What has made you angry lately? If you think about that while watching your face in the mirror, do you see changes?

❧

People can become over-activated within either the sympathetic or parasympathetic nervous system. Sympathetic activation is indicated by increasing energy, or charge. The person may become restless, color may rise, respiration becomes frequent and shallow. This kind of arousal happens when we're excited and when we're scared. When sympathetic arousal gets too high, the person may hyper-focus on stimuli. If arousal continues to build toward the top of the body's tolerance, the PNS kicks in, shrinking visual and auditory perception, slowing the breath, and creating brain fog, pale skin, lassitude, and other indicators. Everyone's ANS has a range of function, and we are always moving up and down in our level of arousal. When arousal gets too high (sympathetic activation) or too low (parasympathetic activation), we can't tolerate or make sense of any new information.

Arousal is observable, as you have just seen with the previous exercise. You can get support for learning to observe from a wonderful chart created by trauma therapist Babette Rothschild (Rothschild 2018). It details observable changes as a person's level of arousal rises and falls. It's a top-down (cognitive) approach that can complement the bottom-up (experiential) learning I'm recommending here, by offering a visual display of the continuum of arousal.

The middle place where our ANS is alert, open to information, and capable of making adjustment is where we are most functional. This arousal window is known as the "window of tolerance." If people get outside that window through over-activation, they often need support to come back into it. We help clients who are over-aroused by too much sympathetic activation to calm by using our calm voice, modeling deeper breathing, inviting attention to the lower parts of the body ("press your feet into the floor"), and asking for eye contact. We help clients come back from parasympathetic over-activation (shutdown) by inviting movement, such as shaking their hands or their heads, and attention to immediate sensory details, such as offering a sip of water.

Mostly, though, our bodies do the heavy lifting of co-regulation, which is particularly important when clients near the edges of their windows of tolerance. Our warm, calm presence, well-modulated voice, clear consistent eye contact, and our own breathing pattern support the client much as she supports her baby with her body. Just as mothers co-regulate their babies' ANS, our bodies help our clients regulate theirs. This is not calculated, just another process variable.

Keeping our bodies stable and regulated throughout a session is key to supporting our client. Not only do we want her well within her window of tolerance, but we'd also like her to be moving toward a stable, social engagement dominant state. That is, we help to up-regulate the dorsal vagal, down-regulate the sympathetic, and up-regulate the ventral vagal so that the ventral vagal part of the ANS is dominant. Sounds impressive and difficult, doesn't it? What it all means is that by being calm, energized, and present to her experience and our own, her nervous system will stabilize and regulate to ours.

More therapist skills: Emotional co-regulation, mirroring, attunement, body resonance

Observation is not the only way in which we share presence with our clients. We have specific interaction skills that increase a sense of presence for both parties and help us (as therapists) grasp more deeply our clients' somatic experiences.

Emotional co-regulation: The need for a therapist to maintain physical calm and stability cannot be overstated. We have already talked about co-regulation of arousal, but your calm presence is also important in regulation of emotion. Your client's emotions may be overwhelming her. She needs to have those feeling experiences in the presence of someone who is not overcome by them. She needs to be with someone who can imagine what it is like to be her, to be inundated but not actually overwhelmed. The client needs to "feel felt" as Siegel (1999) has put it.

When our client is telling us her story, feelings flow. She may want to crush and hide the feelings, but we want to support her in her reality. Ask her about her experience. ("What are you noticing in your body?" rather than "What are you thinking about?") Encourage her to touch the feeling lightly as it arises and then ease away from it. It's a little like dipping your toe into a cold lake. You don't have to keep it there.

There are different ways to do this.

Spiritual teacher Chameli Ardagh suggests the sequence of Feel-Kiss-Flow to help people be with uncomfortable feelings without drowning in them. As the feeling arises, notice the sensations in the body and give them your full attention for a mere moment ("kiss") and then let go. The letting go of attention is gentle and easy, permitting feeling to move and change ("flow"). This sequence helps clients remember that they won't die from their feelings and offers them the control of consciously stepping away. They don't have to shift into defense mode, where they might project, blame or judge themselves. They just step away while the feeling flows.

Trauma therapist Peter Levine (Levine & Frederick 1997) recommends the concept of titration in working with deeply challenging emotional experience. Titration involves balancing support with challenge, helping someone to become accustomed to coping with difficult things. Levine provides steps you can use in this process.

Support your client in identifying her resources, those things or ideas that help her feel better. Her resource can be whatever she chooses: her contact with you, a cognitive reminder ("I can handle this"), a memory ("my dog wagging his tail when he sees me") or a support you simply imagine ("I can see Wonder Woman coming to my rescue"). Invite your client to have a moment of whole-body awareness while she dips her toes into the "yucky stuff." Then pull those toes out, using a resource for support. Since you know what her resources are, you can offer a prompt. Practicing cognitive supports like reminders, positive memories, or imagined helpers makes it more likely your client will use them when she leaves your office.

Titration increases her capacity to tolerate her own feelings. When she practices feeling what she feels with the support of a resource, she increases her tolerance. She experiences her ability to survive her feelings. Increasing familiarity with her sensations and emotions helps her feel safe enough to explore her feelings. As she gains skills in using her resources, she may develop curiosity about her internal process. Titration suggests she can get close to the challenging feeling, then use a resource to step away. Sidle in again and see what it feels like. Then step away and reflect.

Through this sequence, repeated over and over, a woman discovers that she can get in touch with her feelings and survive them. When she increases her emotional tolerance, everyone benefits.

This fear of one's own feelings may sound extreme, but at a very core level, feelings are what we are most afraid of. When we were very small, before we had words, we had very big feelings. Nobody has bigger feelings than a toddler! Some of our feelings were met by our parents and caregivers. Some were encouraged, mirrored, and given space for their expression. Other feelings may have engendered a negative response from the adults around us. Shark music got started there.

Still other feelings may have never been met or met only with absence. This absence of meeting creates an experience in a young mind that is explainable by some failure on the part of the self ("I am too much, I am not enough, I am not worthy, I am unlovable, I don't deserve"). People report, for example, nobody interested in their sadness or fear or being left alone to deal with any big feelings.

The life experience of encountering absence, when what we really needed was presence, is what makes some emotions so impossible to bear in adulthood. Unmet feelings arise in mothers of new babies, who are already in a space where everything seems impossible. These feelings represent the shark music of early motherhood. They magnify everything, and the lack of being met and held and contained in one's own early history shows up with a terrifying familiarity.

When a baby is demanding everything from you, the blank spots in your own emotional experience become painful chasms that you cannot even describe.

Titration allows a mother to feel mastery over overwhelming emotions. Your unflinching presence validates her. Finally being heard can lead to new core beliefs. With your support, she can challenge harsh thoughts, stepping away from believing feeling bad makes her bad, unlovable, or unworthy. Because you, her therapist, can hold her in unconditional regard even when she's feeling and thinking terrible things, she may give herself a chance. Perhaps she's not a terrible person. Maybe she's just a person who is having a very hard time.

This process can feel overwhelming for the therapist. It is okay to feel engulfed momentarily by your client's suffering, a temporary flooding of a boundary (see Chapter 11), but it is not okay to stay there. If you are feeling that way, it does not mean that you are in the wrong field or not a capable professional. It means you need some support. When you feel overwhelmed, it is time for consultation, supervision, and maybe your own therapy. You may find out that there is something cooking for you that you haven't addressed yet. Whenever you are activated by client stuff, it means that you have some of your own emotional processing to do. See Chapter 15.

Mirroring: While we pay deep attention to a client's story and bodily signals, we also mirror their behavior. Mirroring is part of early parenting, but it is also part of everyday interaction. When we mirror another person's behavior, we get to know their somatic experience. We also develop a sense of alignment with them. The other person can feel this alignment too.

How does this work? Mirroring is like an unconscious dance between partners who are in sync. In the context of a deep, curious, compassionate attention, mirroring helps people feel seen. Mothers mirror their babies' facial expressions, amplifying smiles and frowns and giving them words. We see lovers tilt their heads in the same direction. When good friends are having an energized conversation, we can assess their degree of agreement just by watching how much they mirror each other's movements.

Mirroring in therapy helps clients to feel connected to us. Mirroring opportunities includes body positioning, bodily movement, facial expressions, and vocal patterns.

Therapists can quietly adopt the body positioning of the client, noticing how it feels in the body to hold it this way. While our conscious minds are noticing, our neurons and the client's neurons are firing synchronously, creating a feeling (felt sense) of alignment. When the client tilts her head to talk, the therapist tilts to listen.

When a client expresses joy or happiness, a therapist may also look happy. When the client is sad or angry, the therapist is likely to have some facial expression that supports these feelings as well. If a facial expression is incongruent, it may require explanation—"I know you are mad, and my smile is because I am happy to hear the strength in your voice."

Therapists may alter their speech patterns to mirror the way that a client speaks. This is not mimicking or copying but a subtle matching that helps the client to feel connected and that they are okay with you. This is not dissimilar to limiting the use of slang or swear words due to a client's preference.

Experienced therapists do a lot of mirroring without even realizing it. It is a nearly automatic part of relating on a deep level to clients. I watched very experienced EMDR therapist Dr. Mara Tesler-Stein do a demonstration with a participant at a training workshop. At every moment, Dr. Stein was using her whole body to mirror and attune to the client's energetic and emotional flow. When I pointed out the skillful way that she used mirroring, she was surprised as it was simply part of her interaction.

Attunement: This is another "mothering" skill that therapists can learn. Attunement refers to matching the intensity of an expression but doing it in a different modality. A client may say something harsh and angry, and a therapist might say, "Yeah!" and punch her fist into her palm. Similarly, when a client is sad the therapist slows her movements to attune with the feeling state. Attunements often happen spontaneously, especially with experienced therapists. Somatic therapists know that attunements are powerful interventions on their own.

Body resonance: Bodies resonate to each other. We are aware of the ways in which bodies resonate when people live together. We know, for example, that women who live together will coordinate their menstrual cycles. We know that family biological rhythms will become everyday experiences for children (once parents live through the no-sleeping stage). Lovers resonate, in the sense that their bodies generate a response in one another by mere presence.

Somatic therapists can use body resonance for information. We learn to be attentive to our own ongoing flow of somatic experience as we interact with our client. We notice what calls for our attention in our own bodies while we are with her. Then we ask, is this mine? We hold awareness of our own flow while we are with the client, noting her experience simultaneously.

You might wonder how on earth a somatic therapist can hold so much information at once and still do therapy. Perception happens in an instant. We experience it all in a heartbeat and easily focus on our client. After all, she is the reason for our self-awareness. We use all possible sources to help us support her emotional and energetic process.

CHAPTER 6

Using Somatic Interventions

Your skills in therapeutic presence, tracking energy, and titration, detailed previously, will help you in the therapy process. Noting your own somatic process as you sit with clients is a great beginning step. If you are already doing that, congratulations on keeping a high level of self-awareness while working.

Self-awareness isn't the same as self-consciousness. Instead, it is a component of presence. When we are self-aware, we can also be aware of how we are influencing our clients. Tracking alerts us to over-activation, when the client may require co-regulation.

Somatic activities support going deeper into one's immediate experience. This can be activating, and so we monitor. Encouraging small steps helps keep our client within a window where she can process new information, and those small steps are meaningful and more accessible than big changes. We follow each step with reflection. The reflective moment is when the client can integrate the new experience into her existing structure.

Compassionate curiosity plus non-judgment

Somatic therapy teaches us and our clients to slow down and notice what is right here, right now. As a therapist, I'll watch my clients carefully. I am not judging, just noticing. I also must remember that she's the expert on her internal experience. I can never know her inner life. I can, however, be deeply interested in her and invite her to share that space with me.

Imagine your super-power is compassionate curiosity. Bring that to bear as you observe and listen to your client.

Watch for movement in the body. How does she choose to be in your space or in the virtual therapy space? Does she sit facing you directly? Does she curl up and wrap her arms around her knees? In a virtual session, clients choose their own location. Does she have her session with you from her bed? From her car?

Small movements can hold meaning. Watch for

ANS Over-Activation

Over-activation means that the client cannot effectively process her experience. If the client is out of her window of tolerance, her capacity for processing drops. The window of tolerance is a useful concept developed by Dan Siegel to describe the range of autonomic functioning that is optimal for processing information. If we are overactivated by the sympathetic nervous system, or hyper-aroused, we don't function optimally. If we are under-aroused by an overactive PNS, we're also unable to process. We need to help our clients stay in and even expand their personal windows of tolerance. When we help the client to regulate her ANS back into her window of tolerance, we help to stay present to herself and to us. This aids her healing.

characteristic movements. Does she pick at her face? Wring her hands? Sit perfectly still? Move only when talking or move only when you are talking? Just noticing the patterns can be helpful. There is no need to understand, label, or judge them. They simply reflect the somatic reality of your client.

Watch for changes in respiration. Notice how your client is breathing while she is telling her story. Where does her breath create movement? Notice if there are places where she stops breathing and where she takes a deep breath. Take a deep breath yourself and see if she shifts her breathing. When she becomes distressed, what happens to her breathing? Keep watching and noticing.

Watch for skin color changes. Some people overtly register changes in body energy in the skin. Very fair-skinned white people will often become flushed when agitated. People of all skin colors exhibit changes that are related to energy flow. Some are easier to see than others. Faces flush or pale depending on the level of arousal. Other parts of the body also will have color changes related to the capillary blood flow of the moment. Beyond that, parts that feel numb will often look flat and dead, without life, much as frostbitten skin might look. When a body is highly energized, such as after exercise or after kicking, you can observe places where the flush does not seem to flow. You can infer some tension in those places.

Watch for eye contact and the specific quality of eye contact. Pay attention to eye contact: does the client look at you or away from you? Under which circumstances would eye contact occur? Bioenergetic therapists also look at the quality of contact that the person engages through the eyes. Does she seem available for contact? Or is she far away or even unreachable? See if you can look at each eye separately. You may develop some impression of difference between them.

Notice the timbre of the voice. Your voice is a production of a complex system of brain and nervous system and tissues of the throat. It is influenced by the state of your ANS and your emotional state. You have certainly experienced being unable to speak due to strong emotion. Listen to your clients as they tell their stories. You will hear places to follow up around deep feeling because there will be a catch in the voice, a thickening or constriction. You can also notice what words might be hard for your client to say. The process of listening to one's own thoughts spoken aloud is a powerful releaser for emotion. Your presence while she tells her story also helps release the feelings.

Somatic interventions vary in complexity, but even the simplest trains skills in attention and regulation that are helpful for all. I've divided them into three categories. Exercises for each are in the following chapters.

First: Attention to the body

The first level skill we encourage is simple attention to sensations, which we might refer to as "mindfulness of the body." By attending to body sensations before they become alarms, we can better manage what becomes uncomfortable. We teach our clients how to do this through slowing down and redirecting attention. In our sessions, we attend to the sensations reported by the client, while modeling openness and compassionate curiosity.

Second: Grounding and focusing

The next level is grounding and focusing energy. These skills mobilize resources that the client already has, which will help her manage her reactions. After practicing attention, grounding, and focusing, help her stay connected to her somatic experience rather than falling into problem thinking. Practice will change the neural wiring, adjusting her default pattern of self-shaming. This creates space for self-compassion and self-acknowledgment. Grounding helps people feel themselves with less distraction.

Knowing oneself deeply, from a compassionate and friendly stance, expands the range of emotional experience and expression. It creates opportunities for pleasure and enjoyment, which are often in short supply for perinatal clients. The therapist teaches and models these exercises while taking an active role in supporting the client to self-discovery.

Third: Emotional intelligence

The third level skill includes emotional awareness, containment, and expression. Our emotional lives are often truncated and limited. Most people are more interested in controlling their emotions rather than feeling and expressing them. When a woman allows herself to feel what she feels and has wholesome and functional ways to express her feelings, she finds life more satisfying.

Most people had early experiences of being shamed, dismissed, punished, or shunned while having strong feelings. Think of a child being isolated for an angry outburst. Many people are nearly phobic about emotional expression, fearing the abyss of (assumed) social judgment and self-negation. The bigger the feelings, the bigger the fear.

We are most phobic about anger. In our society, anger is regularly weaponized. Anger is used to take and keep power over others, to do harm to others, to elevate oneself above others, to incite others, and to discharge overwhelming agitation. We should be afraid of the misuse of anger.

Unfortunately, we take a shortcut and become afraid of anger itself.

Anger is just a normal emotion. It is normal to feel angry sometimes, just like it is normal to be happy, sad, or afraid. Our emotions convey information. Anger indicates a boundary violated.

Women's anger is a special case. Patriarchal society is quick to ridicule and dismiss women for anger. It's no wonder many women repress or suppress their anger, sometimes to the point that they miss the buildup of intensity, and it emerges as raging. Such outbursts are terrifying, shameful, and overwhelming to both the woman and her family. If she can get to know her anger and learn how to express it in a safe, supported way, she can prevent damaging outbursts.

It requires a solid foundation in body attention, grounding, and focusing to move into practicing emotional expression in therapy. With a therapist who is herself attentive, grounded, and focused, a client can practice moving from expression to reflection, and back again. For example, expressing her anger through twisting a towel, or hitting a pillow, reflecting on the experience, then choosing whether to express further.

Attention, grounding, focus, and fluid movement between expression and reflection are skills. Developing these skills allows our clients to avoid the back-and-forth of rigid control and explosion. A therapist invites expression of all a woman's emotions, helping her to explore expression in a safe and comprehensive way. There is less internal conflict when feelings and behavior match. This internal congruency feels good. Even when uncomfortable feelings arise, they are just feelings.

This congruency allows for acceptance of all feelings. If she is exhausted and overwhelmed, she's exhausted and overwhelmed. It is just how she feels. There is no need of a story of shame and guilt. Strengthening her sense of self opens her to use her body expressively to manage her energy. When she can attend, ground, focus, and express herself, she'll have tools for all sorts of life challenges, for the rest of her life.

How to practice the exercises

The following chapter includes exercises for you to do yourself and with clients. It bears repeating that you need to experience these exercises yourself before adding them to your therapy repertoire.

For each exercise, follow this sequence:

- Check in with your inner space.
- Give yourself time to allow the experience to unfold.
- Take a long moment to note how the process settles in your body.
- Add a note to your journal, detailing your somatic process. What was that exercise like today?

CHAPTER 7

Attention to the Body

Paying attention sounds so simple. We are habituated to paying attention to our surroundings, to things outside us. When I ask clients to simply "notice your breath," sometimes they cannot do it with ease. Becoming aware of what is happening in the body can create a profound shift in how a person relates to their social environment.

This is a very short chapter, but body awareness is fundamental to all the other exercises in the book. Don't let the brevity make you think it is unimportant! Every single exercise will ask you to check in on yourself.

Your clients may initially be surprised that you care about their body sensations, but sensations are the building blocks of feelings, and of course you do care. It helps if you're well acquainted with the range of sensations available in your own body. When I started to do bodywork, I discovered I had been living with low-level belly pain probably forever. I dismissed it, ignored it, and just went on with my life. When I became aware of the pain, I also became aware of how it related to my irritability and lack of patience. I had been completely unaware of this connection.

Try this out and see what you discover.

Exercise #7A: Body Awareness – Interoception

Stand on a carpet or yoga mat for these exercises to cushion your feet without creating a soft surface. Do them barefoot or with socks if your feet are cold. The same instructions apply to clients.

Begin by assuming the orienting position: stand on the floor, feet under your hips, knees soft, head balanced comfortably on top of your spine, and eyes open. From here, you can orient to the room and any available stimulation—sounds, smells, sights. You can also orient to your own body, feeling how you are present in the space. Take the orienting position and check in. Notice your space. Then turn inward. This is the starting place. What do you sense in your body?

Remember that your body takes a bit of time to share information. Give yourself a few moments of sensing and feeling, letting your awareness increase. If your mind has an answer right away, that's okay, but keep inviting your body to offer information. If your mind (or your client) answers with a concept or an emotion (I feel anxious), check in for sensation. (Where do you notice it? What's it like?) You're aiming for the level of sensations here.

What parts of your experience attract most of your attention? If you have been reading or thinking hard, you might notice much of your feeling is in your eyes or your head. You may notice your body more if you have just risen from a sitting position. Do a brief scan to see what parts of you are seeking and receiving the most attention right now.

Now start at your feet and work your way up, noticing whatever there is to notice. Pay attention also to parts of your body that are less easy to access. Your general awareness of your body is your pre-grounding baseline. The next exercises will explore how you ground and how you feel when you are more grounded. You can check later to see if your body awareness has changed.

Take some time to jot notes about what you notice. You could even sketch out a body and mark the places you felt something. Date your notes for your own future reference.

Exercise #7B: Checking In (Short Version of Exercise #3)

Check in with your body any time. In other words, take a mindful/ bodyful moment. Stop what you are doing and allow your attention to turn inward. It's often easiest if you float inward on your breath. Just notice where the breath goes in your body and then let your attention wander around in all those parts. Hang out there for three breaths, or maybe more if you have the time or find something interesting.

Why are you doing this? It's about developing a practice of seeing "how am I now?" Clients report becoming suddenly rageful or impatient, but often it's because they don't notice the early body cues of arousal and distress. Minor pain doesn't get attention until it flares up, but perhaps a well-timed rest could have prevented a flare. Learning to check in with yourself is a simple, low-stakes practice that can pay off in terms of overall comfort and self-knowledge.

To do it, again, follow your breath into body sensations. Just notice whatever you notice. You don't need to change anything, judge anything, do anything. Just breathe and notice. Breathe again, allowing your attention to stay in your experience. And one more breath.

That's all.

Exercise #8A: Self-Touch

Use touch to heighten body awareness.

Stand in the orienting position and take a breath, allowing your attention to move inside. Allow yourself a moment to scan your body for a check-in. Make a gentle note of whatever you notice.

Now place the palm of one hand on the opposite forearm. Grasp your forearm with a comfortable firmness. Notice what it is like to feel your arm in your hand and also to feel a hand on your arm. Then pat or lightly slap up your arm from wrist to shoulder, continuing for a few breaths. Let that movement come to an end. Take a moment to notice each arm. Is your awareness of your arms different? Then slap or pat the other arm, creating a similar awareness.

Continue with using your hands to touch your legs: pat, slap, or stroke your legs, noticing how that affects your awareness of your legs. What other parts of your body are calling out for this kind of attention?

Exercise #8B: Self-Touch Towel Variation

Sit in a chair fully clothed but barefoot, then grasp the ends of a hand towel and loop it under one foot. Briskly tug it back and forth, massaging the arch of your foot. Then slide the towel up the back of the leg, rubbing behind the knee, then around to the front of the thigh, rubbing back and forth as if you were drying off after a shower. Do the same for the other leg.

Loop the towel around your arm and hold the two ends in the other hand. Tug and pull the towel up your arm, again like you are drying off. Repeat on the other side.

Loop the towel around the back of your neck and rub it briskly. Open it up and slide it up the back of your head, against your scalp and over the crown of your head. Notice how your body responds to this attention and touch.

Grasp a palmful of the towel and sweep it across your forehead, around your eyes and down your cheeks. Lightly stroke your face, jawline, and neck. Check to see what other parts of your body want the attention of the towel and accommodate where that is possible.

When you are finished, drop the towel and tune into yourself. What do you notice now about your body awareness?

Exercise #9:   Movement to Heighten Awareness

Lie down on your back in a comfortable position. Use what you need to allow your body to relax. This might include support for your head or neck, a rolled-up towel under your knees, or a blanket over you for warmth. Once you are settled in, lie still, just noticing your breathing.

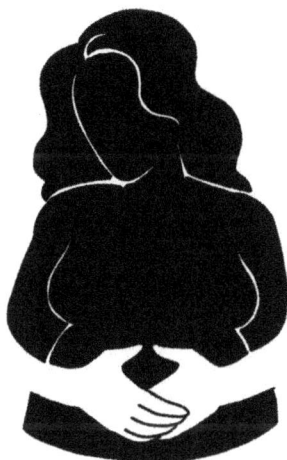

Now think about your toes, bringing them into your field of awareness. After a moment, wiggle them and check again. How did that movement affect your awareness?

Return to stillness. Now bring your fingers into awareness. Without moving them, check to see how aware you can be of your fingers. Then wiggle them.

Return to stillness for a few breaths, then scan your body. Are there parts that are out of awareness? Parts you cannot clearly experience this way? See if there is some movement or touching that brings that part into awareness. Perhaps your low back is a blank spot in awareness. Press it against the floor, massaging it lightly, and see if you are more able to access it.

For each movement you choose to try, take a long moment of reflection to explore what you noticed and how awareness changed.

CHAPTER 8

Grounding: Finding Home Base

Grounding is a concept with a long history, including connections to the ancient practice of tai chi, other early martial arts, the Hindu practice of yoga, and earth-oriented spiritual practices. In general, being "grounded" is the opposite of feeling like you are flying to pieces or like you are "all up in your head." With increasing groundedness, one has a keener sense of body awareness.

Grounding is a continuum. In practical terms, that means we can always become more deeply grounded. Helping a client to increase her grounding is never the wrong intervention in therapy. It involves moving the body to increase the experience of contact with the ground. You may start with your feet on the ground, but after doing grounding exercises you will feel more of the foot-to-ground connection.

Human beings are essentially terrestrial creatures: we are ground-dwellers, most secure when our feet are connected to earth. Birds, monkeys, and squirrels are different. While many humans adapt to flying, it is a special activity for us rather than our everyday way of being in the world.

Grounding exercises stimulate ventral vagal activation. People may yawn deeply as they begin to let down, spontaneously deepening their breathing. Body parts will soften; postural alignment improves without effort. Eyes become softer and, simultaneously, vision may improve. Increasing the sense of being grounded mitigates free-floating anxiety.

Grounding is a concrete body experience. It is a physical experience of our bodies in contact with the environment which affects the flow of energy in the body. As energy flows, sensations, feelings, and thoughts also flow. But when we focus on the movement of the body against the ground, we literally ground the experience, so it is not ethereal or disembodied. It is firmly somatic.

Grounding is completely physical. You will notice changes in your cognitive space while you do grounding exercises, but they are a by-product rather than the thing itself. You may become more mindful of external or internal stimuli, but that is what happens naturally as you move your attention into the present moment. Grounding is a process of connecting your body to the earth, either through the furniture to the floor to the ground, or more directly, depending on where you (literally!) stand.

Observe what is happening in your body as you do these exercises. See if you notice changes in your breathing, in where your body awareness goes, in the content of your thinking processes, including fleeting images, negative thoughts ("this is dumb"), or anything else. This moment-to-moment self-awareness offers self-knowledge and information for you and your client in a therapy session. Follow along with the directions and keep noticing what is happening within you.

Exercise #10: Grounding through the Feet

The standing exercises are best performed with some padding under the feet. A yoga mat, carpet, or a towel can supply some softness to a hard floor and also some texture to help awaken the soles of the feet.

After experiencing your baseline through awareness in the previous exercises, turn your attention to your feet. While standing, check your heels, the balls of your feet, your toes. Where can you sense the weight of your body? Do you carry more weight on one foot than the other? Don't worry about trying to change this; right now you are just noticing. Take a breath or two while you are checking in on how your weight is distributed.

Variation: Waking up the contours

Stand with your feet about hip width apart, or so that the front part of your hip bone is right above each foot, knees slightly bent.

Standing solidly on your two feet, allow your weight to come to the right so that you are standing on the right edges of both feet. Hang out there for a bit, making sure that your knees are soft. Breathe a few times. Notice how your breath feels as you lean hard on the right sides of your feet. Notice any sensations in your ankles, your shins, your feet. Now pump your knees up and down a bit while you are breathing. You can try coordinating your in-breath with bending your knees and your out-breath while you straighten your legs. Just explore.

Now roll your weight across your feet so that you are standing on the left edges of your feet. Keep your knees bent as you would for skiing and let your feet hold your weight. Hang out there and breathe. Try pumping your legs like before. Give yourself a few breaths here.

Roll back to the right side of the feet and repeat the sequence. See what is different as you do it a second time. What do you notice?

Variation: Waking up the joints

Still standing on your mat, bend one foot at the toes, pressing the bottoms of your toes into the floor. Allow the knee of the standing leg to be soft. Strongly push those toes into the floor, bending them and putting some weight into them. Roll the foot slowly from side to side, so that you put pressure on the big toe and then the other toes in turn. Notice what that is like for you. What does your foot say to you about this? You can deepen the experience by pumping the standing leg and breathing along with that movement.

Lift one foot, then place it down with the tops of your toes touching the floor. This bends your ankle in a different direction and puts some pressure on the tops of your toes as well as stretching the top of your foot. For many people, this direction is less comfortable than the other, but your individual experience is what is important. It is okay to push into some discomfort, stretching just a bit more, but be careful: do not push into pain. These exercises are designed to ease tensions in the feet and open up the opportunity for feeling more, not hurt you. Like a deep tissue massage, there often will be intensity of sensation as the tissues release, but extreme pain is a red flag.

Keep the knee of your standing leg soft and pump along with your breathing.

Once you have worked the toes front and back on one foot, allow that foot to settle on the floor again, and take a moment to feel what it is like to have both of your feet under you. You may experience some relief (notice what relief is like in your body) or some other feeling. Then check on your two feet: can you find any differences between them since doing that work on one side? Notice whatever you notice in your feet, legs, and up your whole body.

You might sense that the other foot wants to be worked too. Whether that is part of your experience or not, do the toes exercise, front and back, for the other foot. Then once again place your feet under you, hip distance apart, knees soft but not bent, and become aware of what you gained from this exercise.

Now that you have done this small but not trivial exercise, notice sensations in your body. What do you sense in your legs? Your hips? Your lower back? How about in your jaw? Oddly enough, the ease that we can find in our pelvic floor as we ground our bodies is often reflected in a shift in how we hold our jaw.

Connecting your feet to the ground often makes other body sensations more available. It's the gift that keeps on giving: the more you do it, the more you get from it. A little can help a person feel calmer, more rational, and more able to tolerate confusing emotional states. Doing it regularly can help a person to stay stable during difficult circumstances, manage problem thinking, and feel more like oneself. Being deeply grounded is our natural state.

While you practice, you maintain your ongoing perspective of curious, kindly interest in your own body sensations, accepting everything you perceive as okay. When a mother can trust her own experience of her feet on the ground, she is having a moment of self-trust. She feels what she feels and knows what she knows.

Grounding exercises can be done anytime, anywhere. This work tends to calm sympathetic arousal and activate the social engagement system (ventral vagal). Once you have learned how to connect to grounding through your feet, you can do it on the fly.

Exercise #11: Grounding by Stamping the Feet

Anyone with small children knows about foot stamping. As an adult, though, you might not be aware of how good it can feel and how grounding it can be. The exercise is simple and just as it sounds: stamp your foot on the ground. Pad the floor with a yoga mat or towel if that gives you a chance to stamp harder. Push your foot right down, then lift your knee and do it again. You can work with one leg while the other leg grounds through supporting you. Keep your attention on your body as you work through this process. Hold on to a chair to help balance if that feels better.

Move to the other foot. Once you have fully experienced each foot, try alternating feet while you stomp. Let your arms swing and your eyes flash. Let your body get "into the swing" of stomping your feet, all the while noticing what comes up for you in terms of body sensations, thoughts, feelings, and impulses. When you feel like you've done enough, allow the movement to come to stillness and take the orienting stance, feet under hips, knees soft.

Notice what you got from that activity. Check your connection to the ground. How aware of your feet are you?

Foot stamping with children can be fun and energizing, and it can also provide everyone a bit of relief from tension. Getting more connected to the ground is never a bad thing, and practice in getting charged up and then moving into stillness, especially while noticing how your body feels, is helpful.

Exercise #12: Using an Object on the Feet

Grounding can be facilitated by foot massage. You can effectively massage your foot by rolling it over a tennis ball, lacrosse ball, or even a dowel. Stand in the orienting position and put the dowel or ball under the toes of one foot. Keep the knee of your standing leg soft and let some weight sink over the ball or dowel. Really sink into the feeling at the point of contact. Then roll the ball or dowel back a little and sink in again. Give time in each place for the tissues of your foot to respond to the pressure. You can vary the pressure by varying the weight you put on your foot, and you can moderate the intensity. The intense sensation comes because of tension in your foot; a relaxed foot will easily drape over a dowel or tennis ball. Work your way very slowly on one foot, toes to heel, and back again. Then remove the object and stand on both feet and notice what you notice.

Do your feet feel the same? Is something different? What exactly can you sense?

Now repeat on the other foot. Notice your breathing and how you hold your body as you do the exercise. Note where you want to hurry up and get it over with and where you feel like hanging out and enjoying it. See how your body responds to the intensity of sensation in this exercise.

Standing on both feet after doing this kind of work can be a relief. What a pleasure to have two feet under you! And your connection to the ground may have changed. Notice what that connection is like and whether you can feel any difference in your body or your thinking processes.

Other grounding exercises

These "more advanced" grounding exercises are mostly variations on a theme. You can choose grounding techniques based on your client's preferences, but it is often helpful for people to know several ways to the same end. Clients can explore and decide for themselves what is helpful, and of course bodies are not the same from day to day.

Exercise #13: Forward Bend (Waterfall)

The classic bioenergetic "grounding" exercise is the forward bend. Stand with your feet about hip distance apart, knees soft. Take a moment to notice your feet on the ground, your knees and hips over your feet, and your back, shoulders, and neck. Just notice without judgment.

Drop your head forward and keep dropping it slowly until it takes your body all the way over. "All the way" will be different for different people and may even be different for you from day to day. Let your head, shoulders, and upper body hang over loosely from your hips. Give your head and shoulders a little shake to check and see how loosely you are holding your body. Just hang out here for a bit, breathing and noticing what this feels like.

Now check to see what's going on with you. What has happened in your knees? If they have become rigid, see if you can soften them. See what that brings to you.

Be aware of your hands—you may want to do something with them other than just let them hang but see if you can notice that impulse before moving on it. Let your fingertips just brush the floor so that all your weight rests on your legs and feet.

Keep checking to see if your neck is relaxed and your head is hanging.

Bend and straighten your knees to activate your muscles. When you straighten, push from the floor, keeping knees soft. You can bend as deeply as you like. When you straighten, be aware of pushing your lower back toward the ceiling and hold there for a few breaths. Notice the effect that this movement has on your body. Repeat to see how it changes.

You may feel vibration in your legs and feet. Vibration is your muscles' normal response to working and reflects energy moving in your body. It is not "shaking" in the sense of being uncontrollable. It may be quite pleasant, even if it is unfamiliar, and it can help move feeling through your body. You can easily stop it, or you can encourage it to grow.

You may feel some discomfort in your legs because they are doing quite a bit of work. Can you notice that discomfort and be present to it? The pain of tension because your legs are working is a "clean" pain, one that isn't causing harm and simply reflects effort.

While you are hanging over, make the sound that your legs would make if they had their own voice. Maybe it will be a long groan or a sigh. Make the sound last a long time, as you exhale, and notice if there is any change in the intensity of sensation. You can also rub your calves with your hands or make fists and lightly pound the muscles of the calf as you stay in the bent-over position. Notice what effect that has on the intensity of sensation.

When you have fully explored this exercise, or if five minutes have passed, you can begin to stand upright. Give yourself time to come up very slowly, almost as if you are stacking one vertebra on top of another. Allow your head to hang over until the very last. When you are fully upright, notice what it feels like to reorient.

Take a breath or two and sense how it feels in your body to be standing up after being bent over for so long.

Now turn your attention to your feet and check on your connection to the ground. What do you notice? What parts of your body feel very fresh and clear in your attention right now? What has changed? What is the same?

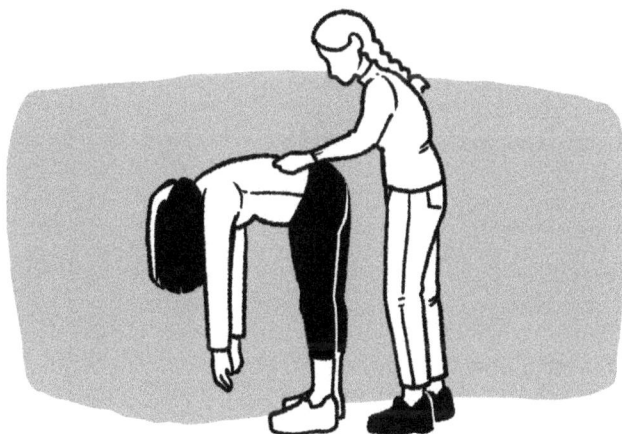

The above exercise has many names, including the forward bend, the bend-over, the waterfall, and the hang-over. It is not a forward fold as we learn in yoga, because it does not ask us to bend tightly from the hips. This exercise can accommodate many body types, because how you hang over will vary with your body configuration. The important factors are to have your legs support you without being rigid and to release the upper body.

You can also explore different ways to hang over: try remaining close to your legs, leaning away from your legs, setting your feet in different positions, and putting your hands on the floor or on your thighs. Notice what you experience from each of these variations. How does your body become most grounded? Can that change from day to day?

Exercise #14: Using the Wall

Having a wall available in your office means that you can invite clients to practice the "wall sit," an exercise that is often used athletically and so may be familiar. The bioenergetic use of the wall sit is different than the athletic version. Rather than building strength and endurance, you're interested in how a person relates to the body experience of being under slight strain while supported. As with any of these exercises, therapists need to have experience and comfort with this before inviting clients to try.

To "sit on the wall," stand with your back to a flat wall, a couple of feet away, bare feet firmly positioned on the floor. The distance of your feet from the wall will vary, depending on how long your thighs are.

Put your back against the wall and bend your knees so that you are "sitting" down as deeply as you can without discomfort. Make sure your sacrum (lower back) is flat against the wall and that you can see your toes past your knees. Settle into the position and allow your breath to deepen. Notice what you are feeling in all parts of your body.

Notice especially your contact with the ground and with the wall. Are you able to let the ground and the wall hold you?

When this begins to feel like "too much," allow yourself to slide up the wall about an inch. Hang out there, breathing and noticing, until that feels like "too much." Then slide up again. Continue hanging out and sliding up until you reach a place where it isn't "too much," and you can feel fairly comfortable in this somewhat strenuous position. Keep breathing and notice your contact with the ground and with the wall.

After some time, you'll be ready to step away from the wall. Move slowly and notice what you experience in your lower body. Then allow your upper body to flow over like a waterfall into the forward bend. Experience that big change in position and stress. Just notice whatever happens.

Strenuous work like this often will tug on memories. Allow yourself to notice whatever arises even if it doesn't make sense.

Flexible boundaries allow others to come close yet are strong enough to limit contact as needed. Working with the somatic aspects of boundaries can bring surprising insight. An explicitly body-oriented approach to boundary awareness provides tools for a lifetime.

Grounding exercises to use while lying down

Exercise #15: Constructive Rest

Lie on your back on a carpet or mat on the floor. You can use a bed if you must, but a firm surface lends itself better to grounding. Let your legs lie flat, arms at your sides, and just take a moment to breathe in this position. If your lower back or knees are uncomfortable flat, use a folded towel to create a little lift behind the knees.

Notice the parts of your body that are touching the floor. Just note what is touching and what is not.

If you can stay in rest for at least five minutes, you will notice some changes in what is touching. Even without thinking about it, your body will start to let down into the ground. Notice what happens in body and in mind as you rest with support.

How difficult is it to allow yourself to rest deeply? What does your mind make of this exercise? This is an excellent exercise for daily practice.

You can end here or go on to the next exercise.

Exercise #16: Grounding through the Feet While Lying Down

From the constructive rest position, bend your knees and allow your soles to come to the floor. Have your feet hip distance apart and a little away from your buttocks. Breathe there and notice what is happening in your body now. Press your soles into the floor as you inhale. Relax with the exhalation. Do this for 10–12 breaths or more. You could go on for a very long time.

Continue until you are ready to end the exercise. As you slow the movement, notice the changes in your body. What are you aware of? What is new after making this movement? What does your body want to do now?

Take your time in getting up. Pay close attention to your experience of moving from horizontal to vertical, from grounding to standing. What do you notice when you are back on your feet?

Getting on the floor can be a great reliever of immediate distress. Getting down on the ground helps us feel our whole bodies, and for most people that is comforting when thinking carries us away. It's also a fun exercise you can teach mothers to do with their babies and children.

I have worked with many clients while sitting on the floor. Often this happens spontaneously because they are caring for babies on the floor, but when a person feels quite frightened, sitting on the floor helps them to be more grounded in reality. Back support helps here. In my office, clients can sit in front of the couch or lean into a supported yoga ball. I also have a supply of pillows that we can use to tailor support to their needs.

CHAPTER 9

The Abdomen in Perinatal Therapy

Culturally we have a lot of unrealistic expectations for our midsections. We idealize the flat belly or the "six-pack abs," but neither of these is very likely for a new mom. Most people have bellies that are overly tight and held-in or are loose and uncontained because of weak muscles. People who have recently given birth have bellies that have been through a lot and need a lot of love.

Having a relaxed belly allows for a full flow of air, and it permits feelings to rise from the lower abdomen into awareness. We are familiar with the idea of the "belly laugh" as a deep, spontaneous movement of the lower abdomen. Adults often cut off their belly laughs, but you can perhaps remember being a kid and laughing so much that you felt like you could not stop. Maybe you even laughed so hard that tears came into your eyes. This is a powerful form of energetic discharge that feels great. It also requires a soft belly.

Deep crying comes from the same area of the body. While laughter is associated with joy or happiness, sobbing and crying are associated with sadness, but the behaviors of laughter and sobbing are very similar and can flow into each other. This is a normal process of discharging the energy of strong emotion. Keeping the belly tight and limited is another way that we keep ourselves from feeling.

Freezing or deadening in the pelvis can happen when a woman struggles with fertility. She may have experienced painful procedures or losses. Even the monthly loss of a period when she wants to be pregnant can be felt as a deadening in the pelvis. Softening the belly can help her open to more feeling and connection to herself.

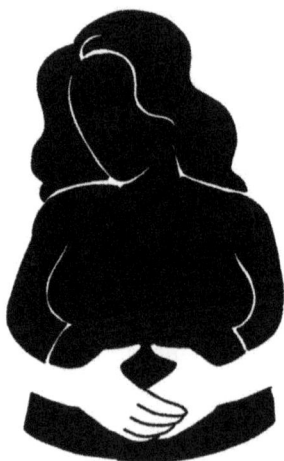

Exercise #17: Awareness of the Belly

Standing or lying on your back, focus your awareness on your belly. Can you feel if you are holding tightly there? Notice any thoughts you have about your belly and bellies in general. What words come to mind? What do you associate with a tight, firm belly? What do you associate with a soft, relaxed belly? This helps you to get a sense of what history you are bringing to the exercise.

Now allow yourself a soft, relaxed, easy feeling belly. Use your hand to rub it in a circular motion, applying gentle pressure to help the muscles relax. How does that feel? Try paying attention from both directions: notice how your abdomen feels to your hand, and also notice how your belly feels from the inside.

Belly rubs are not part of everyday experience for most people, but for a dog, a belly rub might be a bit of heaven. Channel your inner canine to see if you like belly rubs too. These rubs help to activate the PNS, bringing calm, allowing the breath to deepen and tension to ease. Give yourself a few minutes of hands-on belly work to see what it is like for you.

The next exercise is a nice add-on.

Exercise #18: "I Love You" Massage

If you have a little more time, try the "I love you" abdominal massage. Lying on your back, use your hand to trace your lower ribs, your left hip bone, your pubic bone, and your right hip bone. This is the bony framework that holds your abdominal organs, including organs of digestion, elimination, and reproduction. Take a moment to think about the functions of these parts of your body. All sorts of critical things happen within the belly.

Now touch just under your left ribcage and draw a gentle stroke down your abdomen to the left hip bone. Repeat this soft touch on the skin of your belly about ten times. This is the "I" in "I Love You." Now put your fingers under the right ribcage and draw them across your abdomen to the top of the I shape you drew before. Then draw your fingers lightly down again toward your left hip bone. This is the "L" part of the "I Love You" massage. Repeat about ten times, across and down, across and down.

Keep breathing and noticing how you are feeling. The final step is the "U" in "I Love You" and this is done by letting your fingers start in your lower right abdomen just under your hip bone, then gently drawing up to the right ribcage, across to the left ribcage, then down to the left hip bone. (From the vantage point of your head, it is an upside-down letter U.) Repeat this stroke about ten times. This is the "I Love You" massage. You can find videos of this massage on the internet.

This gentle, fingertip manipulation can ease abdominal discomfort and help relax the body all over. It helps support digestion too. For a woman who has become disconnected from her body, especially her abdomen, the "I Love You" massage can be a way of reconnecting to her internal parts.

Increasing connection to the belly

When a woman dissociates from her abdomen, she is missing an important part of herself. Our bellies are the seat of our creativity, not only in reproductive terms but also in the sense that our selves reside somewhere in there. We have gut feelings, and we will often "go with the gut" to make decisions. These metaphors are based in the body because that is where we associate many of the functions of our being. Our bellies have things to tell us. Women who are angry with their bodies are often very angry with their bellies, feeling like they have been let down in the fruition of a long-desired plan.

This body distress is a matter of ego injury, different from feeling "unattractive." For people who have had trouble conceiving or had pregnancy losses, the connection to the body, especially the belly, may be frayed. When a woman is actively frustrated and angry with her body, the idea of sexual pleasure—or any somatic pleasure—becomes foreign.

Being a therapist, as we all know, confers no immunity from struggle. When the issue is a body issue, somatic psychotherapy can be especially helpful.

Case Example #3: Shelly's infertility story

Shelly came in because she was struggling to get pregnant, and she was unable to identify why she was feeling so numb. Shelly was a therapist herself and well-versed in how thinking can become distorted and affect how a person feels.

Shelly talked about her struggles to make appointments at the fertility clinic, her anger at the process of starting with IUI (intra-uterine insemination) when she was sure that IVF would be needed, and how difficult it was to talk with her husband about any of her experiences or thoughts.

Her breathing was shallow as she spoke in the office. She seemed emotionally detached as she clinically detailed her experiences of loss when her period came. She talked about her feelings as if they were happening to someone else.

A few sessions into the therapy, we talked about her body and her belly, in particular. She put her hand on her abdomen but could barely feel her hand at all. As she stayed there, tuning in, she noticed the sensation of light pressure but still could not feel the warmth of her hand.

I invite her to breathe into her hand. "What is that like?"

"Yeah, it's like it's not even there," she says, looking at me. "I didn't realize how much I had cut off."

"It's hard, isn't it, when you want something so much," I offer, while her hand continues to rest on her belly. She looks thoughtful.

"Yes, and I think I might be a little angry."

I nod encouragement.

She goes on. "Angry, maybe, at my body for not doing what it's supposed to do. Everybody else seems to be able to do this simple thing." Her voice grows in intensity. "What's wrong with me?"

I nod again. She is getting to the feeling under the numbness. "Of course you're angry," I say, matching her intensity.

She looks down at her belly, hand still resting on it. She begins to rub a little. "It just seems so hopeless. I think I am doing everything right, and it just doesn't work. I don't work. There is something wrong with me." She looks up at me.

Here is one of those choice-points in therapy. I can reassure her, but that is likely to take her out of her experience. Instead, I can be with her hopelessness, anger, and maybe even despair. I can stay close, instead of stepping away and pulling her away from her feelings into thinking. While staying close, I am compassionately curious about her body experience.

"Oh, wow, Shelly," I say, acknowledging the pain and power of her words. "What are you noticing as you say that?"

Tears fall and she presses her hand deeper into her belly. "I want to be okay! I hate this crap of failing every month and feeling so terrible, and nobody gets it, not even Jared (her husband). This sucks!"

"Yes, it does." I mirror her intensity and expression. "It sucks."

"I hate it."

"Yeah."

"I'm just so tired of the whole thing. Sick of thinking about nothing else. Pissed off that I can't even get pregnant, like everybody else." Her hands make fists. Mine do, too, as I mirror her behavior.

The wave of anger abates, and she cries harder for a moment, then pokes around for a tissue. She tries to stop her crying, but I encourage the release.

"Just let that come out, Shelly. It is okay." With tissues in hand, she sobs a few times and more tears fall. I stay connected with her, breathing into my belly. This is the process.

In a few minutes, she also takes a deeper breath and settles into her seat. "I guess this whole thing has been harder than I realized," she says.

"It is very hard," I offer agreement. "How is your belly feeling?"

She puts her hand back on her abdomen. "Hmm. I can feel my

hand now," she reports with wonder.

"Hmm," I say. "What is that like?"

She is still tuned to her internal experience. "Yeah, good, I think. I can feel a little more space in there. I am still mad and sad, but I can feel that. It feels better than just numb. That was a little scary."

"I am glad you are feeling more of yourself now. What do you think you might be able to do to stay connected to that part?"

We move into a discussion about what she can do at home, and she decides to have a long bath twice a week and dialogue with her belly and use a journal to connect her thoughts to her body as she continues in her infertility treatment.

With Shelly, the work was entirely about her body and how she related to her body, and specifically the ways that her fertility status interacted with her ability to feel in her abdomen. She was tightly closed up so that she could not feel much, because the waves of sadness and anger felt like they might overwhelm her. By getting access to her own body experience, she released some tightness through active crying, regaining connection to her feelings.

CHAPTER 10

Breath and Body

Breathing is as involuntary and natural as anything our bodies do. It is the activity that we engage in all the time, waking and sleeping, and it keeps us engaged with the world around us. We take in oxygen, release carbon dioxide, and repeat. It's totally natural, normal, and accessible. It's a great way for clients to practice mindfulness of the body.

Our breathing changes spontaneously with activity and in response to changes in our ANS. When our sympathetic system activates, respiration becomes shallower and lighter. As we settle back down, breathing deepens again. Similarly, when we engage in activities that deepen our relaxation—getting a long warm hug, having a massage, settling down on the couch when the kids have finally gone to bed— our breath becomes deeper.

We can invite our clients to notice their breathing at any time. When we model noticing the breath as they talk, we encourage them to stay in connection with the breath too. Often, our changing respiration is a first indicator of changing autonomic functioning. That is, we might feel like we've stopped breathing within an interaction, and that may precede scary thoughts or worries that arise. Or we might notice how deep the breath goes into the belly as we settle into a hot bath or our comfortable bed. These moments of awareness help us to stay more connected to the somatic realities of our lives and help us to get to know ourselves better.

We have some degree of control over how deeply and fully we breathe. We can even influence our ANS by consciously deepening respiration so that our diaphragms are actively moving as we breathe. It is as if the deep breath and easy flow of the diaphragm tells our ANS "everything's okay." This is the classic "belly breathing" taught in relaxation. It's also useful to therapists who are helping clients with stress or anxiety and a good tool for parents to use with their kids.

Seeing the breath move in the body takes practice. Observe yourself in a full-length mirror, pretending you are a client. Later, try it out on family members. Ask yourself the following questions.

- What can you see as they inhale and exhale?
- Can you see movement in the chest?
- In the abdomen?
- Is there a labored quality to breathing?
- Are there any breath sounds?

The next step is to coordinate your observation with listening. During a conversation, notice the other person's breathing as they talk. Breathing will change as the story is told. This reflects the ways the story affects ANS activation level.

Does her breathing become shallow? If so, her diaphragm is tightening up, not letting the air down. Shallow breathing is associated with sympathetic activation (distress or agitation).

Does her breathing slow and deepen into her belly? These changes suggest movement toward relaxation and release.

Does the client seem to hold her breath? You may see distinct color changes in her skin as the breathing movement ceases. She is probably not holding her breath entirely, or at least she won't be doing it for long, but she has shut breathing down to a minimum. This can be a fear response or an involuntary effort to stop feeling some emotional content.

At times, a client may tighten her shoulders and neck to keep from breathing more deeply. Restricting the breath shuts off feeling quite effectively, usually without conscious awareness. When you observe increased restriction of breathing movement, ask the client to check in with herself. ("What are you noticing right now?") She can then bring her unconscious response into conscious awareness.

You can ask directly too. Aim for a light, friendly tone to encourage her to feel curious and interested in herself and remind everyone there's no way to be wrong here. "What do you notice about your breathing?" you might ask. After all, you don't know what is happening in her breathing. Often, she will take a moment to assess and then comment on what she notices, often with a laugh or note of surprise.

That light and interested tone is important whenever you inquire about a somatic function, but especially with the breath. Perinatal women are prone to self-criticism and sensitive to perceived criticism from others. She may assume judgment where there is none. Alas, breathing is an area that has become performance-based. People assume that there is a "right" way, and of course they are not doing it. I have had many clients who worry that they "don't know how to breathe correctly," which is an unfortunate legacy of some older breathwork programs.

We don't advocate a "right" way to breathe. If you're alive, you're breathing the right way. However, we encourage awareness of one's own breathing patterns because that's part of knowing oneself. Helping clients understand how breathing relates to sympathetic activation develops self-mastery and self-regulation skills. Watching the breath gives therapists information, and learning to increase awareness helps mothers.

Exercise #19: Breath Awareness

Take a moment to notice your own breath. Just a moment, just three breaths long. Don't change anything. Just notice your body breathing.

What was that like for you? Try to do this a few times a day. Choose different times of day when you're involved with different activities. What do you notice?

Quick and easy ways to activate the diaphragm

There are easy and simple ways to help mothers to become better acquainted with their own breathing. Breath awareness heightens body consciousness generally and regulates nervous system functioning.

When people embrace "deep breathing," they often try to take a long, voluminous breath. In fact, this was how we once taught Lamaze childbirth classes. "Take a deep cleansing breath." Often people cannot get in much air on the first try, especially if they are at all agitated or anxious.

The direction to "take a deep breath" is useless for a mom whose diaphragm is locked up in shallow breathing. She cannot take a deep breath, not yet. There is no space for that air to enter.

There is nothing terribly wrong if you, or your client, cannot take a deep breath. The air needs room. Instead of focusing on bringing air in, focus on moving air out. Air out first. Try this yourself.

Exercise #20: Candle-Blowing Breath

Exhale for as long as you can. Better yet, purse your lips like you are blowing out a candle and then pretend that the candle is across the room. Blow out as long as you can and then blow a bit more and then, like a miracle of nature, your body will breathe on its own. Okay, it really is a miracle of nature. Your body breathes by itself, without anyone being in control.

The breath that comes in will be as deep as it can be given the room that you have made by blowing out all the air. Doing this a few times may make you feel a little dizzy, especially if you are typically a shallow breather. Don't worry. You can return to your natural breath whenever you want. In fact, try just one or two of those "candle-blowing breaths" and then check in with yourself. As with all your exercises, check in to see what you got from it. What did you get?

Mothers may need to be reminded that however they are breathing is just fine; it has kept them alive thus far and they don't need to worry about breathing correctly. We all have our natural breath, and we have variations that are available to us that we can explore. If we find that a particular variation feels good, we might practice that for a while. If we find that a particular variation gives us more information about ourselves and our somatic reality, that might be interesting and helpful.

Exercise #21: Belly Breathing

A common misconception is that "belly breathing" is better in some way than other types of breathing. Breathing so that you have movement in the abdomen is a way to ensure that your diaphragm is moving with your breath, and deepening the breath into the belly is likely to be calming to the ANS. It can be a good thing, but it is not the only or always preferred thing. However, learning how to do it is helpful.

A fun and easy way to connect to the breath in the belly is to lie on the floor on your back, weight the belly with a big book (or a baby), and breathe. As you inhale, make that belly bigger. As you exhale, bring the belly back toward the spine. This sounds easier than it is, but it is almost always fun to try, plus it gives mothers a moment to lie down.

This activity can be taught to young children easily once they reach the age of four or five. We have used small beanbag animals as "breathing buddies" to rest on the belly. The direction for the child is to give the breathing buddy a gentle ride up and down as the child lies on the floor and breathes.

You can also do belly breathing in a vertical position. Stand with both feet under your hips with one hand on your belly and the other on your sacrum. When you inhale, "fill" the hand on your belly. When you exhale, allow that hand to move closer to your back (as if it is going through your body). When you explore this way of belly breathing, you may become more aware of the way your pelvis moves during your normal breathing. Our whole bodies are involved in this utterly common miracle of bringing the breath into the body and moving it out. The pelvis will rock subtly as you inhale and exhale.

What do you notice as you attend to your breathing? What do you notice when you return to your normal awareness?

Exercise #22: (FOR THE THERAPIST) Breathing into the Pelvis

Deeper somatic awareness may allow you to notice how your pelvic floor is related to your breathing. Sitting comfortably upright, bring your attention to your pelvic floor, that internal hammock of tissue that supports your organs. Drop your awareness a little lower to your perineum, the part of your body that lies between your genitals and your anus. Notice the pelvic floor and the perineum. Feel into that space and allow it to be in your awareness.

You may not have any words for the sensations, but you can still note them. Then become aware of your in-breath and your out-breath. Notice how those breathing movements affect your pelvis. Just tune in and then ease back a little. Tune in and ease out. Know that however you are breathing, you are alive, and so you most certainly are doing it right.

You can also lie on your back with your feet flat on the floor, knees comfortably bent. If your neck is very tight, you might explore using the rolled-up end of a hand towel behind your head, just to invite your neck to relax. You can also use a flat pillow, if you like, but the idea is to have your spine generally straight.

Take a moment in this position to notice your body. See how you are relating to the floor. Notice if you can allow your weight down into the floor. Notice where your breath flows in your body.

Now put a hand on your lower abdomen and see if you can bring the breath to your hand. Be aware of a gentle rise and fall of your abdomen as you inhale and exhale. You do not have to work hard at this.

Rather, it is simply allowing your breath to move within your body in the way that it wants to flow.

Take time here to notice your pelvic floor. With your feet flat on the floor and knees bent, you can play with moving your knees closer together and then farther apart. Notice any effect that this movement has on your breathing.

When you are ready to finish, allow yourself to roll over on one side and rest there for a moment before coming upright. When you stand up, take time to notice how your body is making the adjustment from being horizontal to being vertical. Take plenty of time to notice your body awareness, what happens to your breathing, and where your thoughts go.

Doing this exercise yourself will help you to identify your own areas of tension and ease, comfort and discomfort, and to notice whatever images, thoughts, and feelings arise. If a lot of feelings come up, you could consider working with a somatically-trained therapist. I do not recommend this exercise with clients unless you are well-trained in body psychotherapy, body work with specific pelvic training, or somatic sex education. However, I think it is highly beneficial to you as a therapist to be in touch with whatever arises from attending to your pelvic floor.

Breathing to calm, breathing to activate

Our ANS, that brilliant neural network that keeps us alive and functioning, maintains our respiration. We can become aware of our own and our clients' autonomic functioning while noting what is happening with breathing, as well as changing breathing to support particular ANS functioning.

Specifically, we can deepen and slow our breathing to calm an overactive sympathetic system. Any of the breathing exercises to activate the diaphragm will help clients to slow and deepen breathing for calming.

It is often useful to count breaths. If you take five breaths, counting them and noting "I am breathing in" on the in-breath and "I am breathing out" on the out-breath, you may subjectively experience a decrease in arousal. This is a very simple and easy strategy to implement. Remember to practice it with your clients rather than describing it. They are more likely to use it if they have tried it in your office.

Deeper and faster breathing energizes the body. People who are exhausted don't move much, so they breathe shallowly and that saves energy. But pumping up the breath can help a body feel more energetic, at least temporarily. Sleep and nutrition matter for long-term energy.

Here is an activating breathing exercise.

Exercise #23: The Joy of Being Alive

We can also use the breath to increase activation. The exercise called The Joy of Being Alive is a good example (Lowen 1977, 2012).

From a standing position, with feet apart, a little wider than your hips, and knees soft, swing the arms forward up above the head, then down and back, coordinating your breathing with the movement. Inhale as you swing up, and exhale as your arms swing down and back. Keep breathing and swinging until you feel a bit charged up. Respiration rate will probably increase but the volume of air may increase as well, dropping into your belly. Keep your feet on the ground as you swing your arms and stretch upward.

When you are ready to finish, allow the movement of your body to slow gradually to a stop. Take a moment in the standing position to notice what effect this exercise had on your body and your mind. What has changed? What do you notice now?

Most people employ helpful breathing strategies, but they may not be aware that they are doing so. Becoming aware of the strategies that they already use tends to help people feel more competent, and of course they are likely to use something that they, themselves, have invented. Drawing attention to any strategies you see your clients use to modify their breathing can help support their sense of agency.

Chapter 11

Boundaries

Our boundaries reflect our sense of self in the world. We have emotional, behavioral, and somatic boundaries—the points of transaction between us and the environment. For example, our skin is impervious to water but slightly porous to air. The membranes that line our lungs are more porous to air than our skin. We inhale air that brushes across our faces but becomes part of our bodies once it enters our lungs. The lungs select oxygen and release carbon dioxide. This is the transaction within the organ itself.

Psychological boundaries are the points of transactions between people. They tell you where you begin and end and what belongs to you and to others. You may have had interactions that feel like you've been run over with a steam roller. This is usually because the other person is pressing hard against your boundaries, causing you to recoil and pull back, flatten out your own energy. You may also have interactions with someone who seems to try to soak you up, sucking away your time, energy, and capacities. This person is pulling you in with their porous boundaries, and you are pressured to hold your own boundaries tightly. Your boundaries are your safety as well as your invitation to connection.

Our bodies are boundary points that contribute to our sense of self, begun in infancy. Some people struggle to feel their somatic outlines. Somatic work helps to reinforce the experience of being in a body and therefore having boundaries.

Boundaries can be limits, and somatic boundaries are often about body contact. Maintaining limits keeps us safe from invasion or being overrun. Strong limits might protect us but also separate us, cutting off intimate connections. Finding the right balance is a life's work. It depends on a complex interplay of your own experiences and those of the other person, plus the demand characteristics of the situation. When stakes are high—there's a new baby, or life-threatening illness, or danger—it affects how we relate to one another. It is no wonder that "boundaries" are always a hot topic in therapy.

Exercise #24: Mapping Body Boundaries

Stand in the orienting position, feeling your feet press into the ground, your torso erect, and your head on top of your spine. Move your arms through the air so that you can feel them. Inhale and notice how the breath moves into and out of your body. Take a moment here.

Now find some support for your back while you are standing. You can lean against a wall, or if you have a big exercise ball, put the ball against the wall and lean your back on the ball. Press right into the ball or the wall. Keep your attention on the parts of your body that are in contact with the wall or the ball.

Move around so different parts are in contact with the solid surface of the wall or the ball. Feel the contours of your back body. Press your feet into the floor and, if you like, put a palm on top of your head and press down lightly. These are the limits of your body—back, top, and bottom.

Now give yourself a break from this. Step away from the wall or ball and take another moment in the orienting position. Breathe and notice whatever is going on in your body. What is it like to step away from that clear contact?

In the next phase, bring a throw pillow or cushion to where you are working against the wall. Return to the supported position, leaning against the wall or ball, feet pressing into the floor, then hold the pillow against your front torso. Hold it with both arms and feel your whole body contained between pillow and wall or ball, floor, and the top of your head. Breathe in this space a few times. Notice how it feels to have those parts of your body so clear in your mind.

If you like, you can add some words. See what arises organically, or you can try out, "This is me."

Allow your body to stay in this position for a few moments, then when you decide to step away, first drop the pillow. Take a breath to notice any changes. Then step away from the wall and take another moment. Notice the transitions between feeling those defining limits and feeling air.

❧

Boundary wounding is a term that means a person has had intrusions or assaults on their sense of self that can leave the nervous system traumatized. Physical trauma from an accident or injury can make people highly vulnerable to re-wounding.

Here's an example. Imagine a person who has been in a car accident, where the impact came from the left rear. Her nervous system learned that danger comes from that orientation, and when her doctor (or anyone) comes from the left rear, she has a big reaction. She has no such response to someone approaching from the right. This discrepancy makes her feel foolish and ashamed, but it's simply a physiological effect of her accident.

Fortunately, we are all learning more and doing better. Trauma-informed care takes such wounding into account, approaching all patients with awareness.

Boundary wounding can also be emotional and psychological. Interactions that leave us feeling open, raw, or endangered can create long-lasting injuries that go unnoticed until we encounter a similar situation. Bullying is, by definition, an intrusion through a boundary. It strikes at the heart of a person's sense of self and can create long-lasting vulnerability that manifests as distrust of entire classes of people (e.g., I don't trust health care workers, I don't trust the police, I don't trust men).

Childbearing challenges boundaries

Just being pregnant is a challenge to some people. I've worked with clients who struggle with the idea that a baby could be inside them, feeling invaded and not like themselves. For most, the integration of fetus and mother feels like a good thing, despite the inconveniences and downright misery some pregnancies entail. The anticipated outcome helps support a woman through a lot of suffering.

However, that's not the only boundary challenge. Our collective consciousness of the importance of childbearing results in other people violating typical social boundaries. Strangers comment on and touch without permission. This can be profoundly uncomfortable for the person on the receiving end. Learning to say a clear "no" to such violations will help her navigate the more difficult limits later.

Her medical care may require flexibility that stretches the limits of comfort. She may have to allow care providers to do internal examinations, as well as frequent measurements of her body parameters. If she has experienced body boundary violations, she may find these touches intolerable. Helping her to identify her personal limits and strategize how to work with those external pressures is often part of the therapist's role.

To further complicate the boundaries picture, in early parenthood the mother will often feel a bodily connection to the baby. The process of birth doesn't automatically confer the feeling of separateness between mother and baby that other people experience in their interactions with the dyad. This may be even more true if the mother is feeding the baby from her body.

When a mother feels her baby as an extension of herself, or even as an integral part of herself, the interest of other people can feel extremely intrusive. Women often create a small circle of care for themselves and the baby. This can include the father, other children, and sometimes her mother or a close friend. Others feel like intruders.

If a woman has been good at setting and keeping limits in her life before the baby, she may be mildly challenged by the intrusions of the postpartum period. If she has practiced "going along to get along," she may find that strategy no longer works.

In the first months, mother-and-baby are a unit, with boundaries existing between that unit and the rest of the world. This has benefits and challenges, of course, as families navigate integrating the baby as a new member who relates with everyone. During this period, the mother is negotiating boundaries for herself and for the baby.

Flexible boundaries allow others to come close at the discretion of the mother and are also strong enough to limit contact as needed. Working with the somatic aspects of boundaries can bring surprising insight. An explicitly body-oriented approach to boundary awareness provides tools for a lifetime.

Body awareness of boundaries and closeness

You can try this exercise with a friend or partner, or use your imagination to bring another person in. I suggest that you try it different ways, just to increase your own boundary awareness. This first version is for you to try. The second version is how to work with clients.

Exercise #25: Boundary Awareness

Stand in the orienting position (feet under hips, pointing forward, hips over ankles, shoulders over hips, head erect on your spine). Ask your partner to stand facing you several feet away. Take a moment to notice your body standing. Check on your grounding, breathing, areas of tension and relaxation, the inevitable thought parade.

Now look at the person across from you. Notice the sensations that arise as you pay attention to that person. Sense the distance between you. Test out eye contact. How does that feel?

How would it be for the person to move closer to you? In order to assess, you might need to break off eye contact. Take a moment to imagine the person coming closer, then ask them to take a step toward you.

Now recheck your experience. What is different now? Just notice what it is, and then ask for another step closer. With each step, pause long enough to allow your body to register the change and notice your own somatic and cognitive responses. Check out eye contact at each position, just to explore how that changes things.

There will be a point that feels like enough. Close enough. You might overshoot enough and find yourself already in "too close." Notice how it feels and then ask the person to move back one step. Check and see what that feels like in your body. If you manage to stop before "too much," ask for another step toward you, just to see if you can find your "too much."

Take a break and debrief with your partner. What was that like for each of you? How did eye contact make a difference in your experience?

Exercise #26: Boundary Awareness without Visual Input

You can explore your boundary awareness all around your body. Ask your partner to explore with you by walking very quietly around you.

Keep your eyes to the front and notice what it is like in your body when a person is walking to your left, your right, and then directly behind.

Can you sense the person's distance from you without seeing them? Let yourself tune into all of your senses. If you notice a feeling of "too close," ask the person to stop where they are. Visually check out the distance. Was that what you sensed? How accurate was your body sense?

Exercise variations: Working with an imagined partner

Imagine a person in front of you as you stand in the orienting position. Take time to imagine them at a specific distance from you. Clearly image their face and body, recall their voice, characteristic ways of moving, typical fragrance, if appropriate. Use all your senses to make this person as real as possible.

Now imagine them walking very slowly toward you. Pay close attention to your body responses as you create this image.

The advantage of using an imaginal person is that you can change people. Try this exercise first with someone you like and trust. Then give yourself space to imagine someone different, with whom your relationship may be more complicated. Are there any differences in your body response to this person? What happens in your body when you imagine them coming closer?

Exercise #27: Boundary Awareness with Clients

Do the boundary awareness exercise with your client just as you did with your partner. Let the client know that she is in charge of how close or how far away you stand. Start as far away as you can get in your office and encourage her to spend plenty of time checking in on her experience of you. Observe how she uses eye contact. Notice your own feelings of contact or distance from the client.

Make yourself available for connection while you stand in front of her but see if you can sense her receptivity. Watch the flow of energy in her as you explore this together. When she has reached her "close enough," stay there for a bit. Does her tolerance increase or decrease as you stay just close enough? Tell her you're going to take a step back and ask her to monitor her experience. Notice what happens there.

Many women have learned to "tolerate" a level of intrusion that doesn't really feel good. She may notice some relief as you step back. If so, you can explore why she was willing to have you so close that it felt like a little too much. Help her to enjoy and appreciate the feelings of relief that may arise.

Some clients cannot feel a place that is "enough," and you might reach your "enough" before she does. Honor your own sense of "close enough." She may be okay with you coming closer, but you might be finished, and that's okay. If she spends a lot of time merged with others, her sense of herself may not be strong enough to support her awareness of self and other. When you honor your own boundaries with her, you are modeling self-possession. You also create permission for her to claim her own space.

Setting limits and firming up boundaries

The process of setting limits challenges a lot of people. Limits are the concrete manifestations of boundaries. Whole books have been published about limit setting because we have a lot of cultural confusion around personal power and sovereignty. Issues of gender, race, and social class play into this as well. When we work at the level of body response, we set aside those category variables and work with direct experience.

The next set of exercises come from my bioenergetic colleague, Laurie Ure. Many people have trouble saying No. We say we "feel" guilty, but the basic question remains. What is it like in your body when you say No?

Exercise #28: Boundaries – Working with Limit Setting

Practice this yourself before trying it with clients.

Start in the orienting position. Take a moment to check in with your body experience of standing, preparing to explore limit setting.

Bend and straighten your knees a few times. Exhale as you straighten. Press your feet into the ground as you push up. Feel your connection to the earth.

Now extend both of your arms forward, hands flexed. Push the heels of your hands away from you, toward the opposite wall. Imagine your hands are actually pushing on the wall. Feel the whole length of your arm from your shoulder blade, down through your straight elbow, right through the heel of your hand. Notice what it is like to push the other wall away.

Narrow your eyes and push with the heel of your hand. See what words form to go with this movement. Say those words and let your voice match the intensity of the push in your arms. Continue pushing away and using your voice and narrowed eyes for a few minutes. You might be saying "No!" or "Back off," or "Get away from me," or whatever arises for you.

Let your arms drop and take a moment to check in. Shake out your arms, if you like, but allow your attention to stay with your process. What does it feel like inside you to push away with your arms, your eyes, and your voice?

Now try the exercise again. This time, explore pushing away all around you. In which direction do you feel the most desire to push away? Above you, to the right or left, near your feet, or behind? Explore all the way around, keeping a strong voice, face, and push in your arms. This is an exploration of your experience of setting limits around your body. When you feel ready to end the exercise, take a few minutes to shake out and ground yourself. Reflect on your process.

When you do this exercise with clients, you can either be the support on the side as she pushes away, or you can embody the person she is setting limits with. In the second case, you would position yourself across from where she is pushing with the heels of her hands.

Exercise #29: Boundaries – Working with Invitation

When we are in possession of ourselves, we can set limits, and we can invite people to come closer. We also have flexible boundaries under our control. It's important to have both modes available. If we only set limits, we can feel isolated and alone. If we let everyone all the way in, we feel overwhelmed and diffuse, unable to find a sense of ourselves. With a strong sense of self, a person can invite others to come in closer without risking loss of self. Good limits mean invitation is possible.

Start from the orienting position. Begin by pushing as you did in the previous exercise, with narrowed eyes and straight arms. Feel the strength in your back, shoulders, and arms. Keep knees soft and feet connected to the ground. Now drop your arms and soften your face. Think about someone you want to invite into your life, someone you'd like to come closer. See if you can bring a sense of that person into your chest. Allow that feeling to expand and gradually extend your arms from the middle of your back right out in front of you. Stretch your fingers out, open your eyes, and allow the feeling of the person you are inviting to spread down your arms and out your fingers.

Imagine you are inviting that person to come closer. Notice what it is like to invite someone in. Notice any sensations along your arms, through your shoulders, into your chest, throat, or belly. What is it like to create an invitation to someone to come closer? Can you extend the sense of invitation into your eyes?

Exercise #30: Variation – Welcoming and Setting a Limit

This exercise helps to clarify the nature of our real-life boundaries with people. Sometimes we want to bring them close, and other times we want them to keep a distance.

Try going from a limit-setting stance to an invitational stance. First, flex your hands and push out with the heels of your hands as you did before. Narrow your eyes, keep your knees soft and feet connected to the ground, and push away. Feel your strength in setting a limit. You might even say "no" or "get back."

Then allow your body to shift to a reaching, inviting stance. Open your eyes, soften your elbows and your hands, and reach through your fingers. Reach with your eyes. You can speak your invitation too, using words like "come here" or "I want you." When you have explored this experience, return to limit setting with strong arms and flexed hands. What is it like to shift again?

Spend time alternating between setting a limit and offering an invitation. Then let your arms rest and take a moment to see what you're experiencing in your body and mind. How was it to switch gears from a clear limit to a clear invitation? What thoughts, images, or feelings came up for you?

In real life we may switch modes rapidly. Try this. From your grounded position, reach out in invitation with one hand. Use the heel of your other hand to set a limit. You can reach out with one hand while you hold the limiting hand close, ready to deploy as needed. You can enforce the limit with your inviting hand closer to you. Notice how that feels in your body. Try extending both hands at the same time, with those different messages. What is it like to bring in and also to limit access? Which feels stronger? Which feels more like you? What would you like to work on?

What was that like for you? Are you more comfortable saying No or saying Yes? How did it feel to reach and set a limit at the same time?

CHAPTER 12

Embodying Emotion

Embodiment means to experience something explicitly and somatically. Many of us live "in our heads" through continuous thinking, lost in the past or the future. Embodiment means bringing those intellectual experiences into subjective experience.

We know about becoming disembodied. We have great skills at shutting down feelings and experiences in the body. We tighten, constrict, cut off our breathing, and do other spontaneous things to keep us from fully experiencing our feelings. We learn to shut down because emotional expression is not welcomed in most social situations. Also, cutting off feeling through tightening our bodies helps us avoid the feeling itself. Most of us can squeeze back tears and cut off angry words, and we rarely hit or kick when other people frustrate us. Sometimes we shut down so well that we cannot recognize our feelings. We learned how to do this when we were very young.

Disembodied emotion

It is true that we cannot behave like toddlers and still function socially. We do need to delay gratification and tolerate frustration; we need to learn how to channel our feelings into action that isn't harmful. Unfortunately, some of us have gone beyond those limits and tried to stop feeling anything. For some people, disembodiment is about daydreaming a life rather than living. Others overwork or dissociate. Some aspire to spirituality, always seeking a higher plane than our messy somatic reality offers. These are all ways to cut off feeling.

Most of us have shut ourselves down to some degree. We may believe emotions are dangerous or that there are "negative" emotions. Neither of these is true. Emotions are neither dangerous nor negative.

There are no negative or positive feelings. Feelings are temporary body states that shift and change quite quickly. Some are pleasant, and we want them to last longer. Some are very unpleasant, and we would prefer to avoid them. Body states arise and subside, much like fatigue, or hunger, or interest. We are not afraid of feeling tired. We know that weariness will come, and it will go.

We might need to rest, or we might not. But we're not afraid or ashamed of it.

Emotions frighten us because we confuse the feeling with behaviors that are associated with it. We are afraid of anger because it can come with violence. It is smart and reasonable to be afraid of violence. But anger is not violence. Anger is a feeling. We don't need to be afraid of a feeling.

When we tighten up to keep our emotions/feelings at bay, we also lose access to our pleasant feelings. A tight, rigid, constricted body does not allow for much pleasure. People who are tightly held don't feel the pleasant flow of energy throughout the body.

When rigidity makes our bodies too small and tight to hold what we are feeling, we risk explosion. Mothers who build up resentment and pressure and then explode in anger have this experience.

As we've established before, emotions are a body experience, but people work hard to try to turn them into something else. They repress, or suppress, or analyze, making up stories about their feelings instead of experiencing them. These strategies just don't work. However, when a person does feel and fully experience their emotions, the story that attaches often becomes more clear, understandable, and rational.

The distorted story is a way to bypass the feeling. If I can blame someone else, or shame myself, I can get lost in the thinking and not notice how I'm really feeling. Inviting the emotion into experience allows processing without the defensive shame, guilt, or projection.

Here's an example.

I have been disrespected by my partner. I asked him to do something, and he completely forgot. He was more interested in the hockey game than what I needed from him. He has no respect for me as a person. I'm furious with him. He says he made a mistake, it's not a big deal, and he's sorry. He thinks I should just let it go. But it will happen again. He doesn't respect me.

With this story, I can feel my anger/annoyance at him. I tell him how I feel. I'm angry because he disrespected me and I don't believe he's ever going to change. He repeats his apology, but I keep bringing it up because it doesn't feel okay. Even though I talked to him about "my feelings," I'm still mad, and I keep on telling myself the story.

There is something else going on here. Something unprocessed lurks under the story and the anger. I blame, he's wrong, I'm right, and nobody is happy.

Allowing time and space to invite all the emotion in allows us to feel below the projections. The anger is there, yes, and disappointment. Disappointment comprises anger and sadness. Is there sadness? And what else? Maybe even despair.

Letting those feelings move in my body may mean hitting a pillow, or crying, or sinking into collapse for a moment. As the process happens, the story often changes. From "you did this to me" I find "I feel this and this and this and I want/need/desire that."

The change in the narrative follows the changes in the body process. But that isn't a goal. Our only goal is to offer processing space and time for the feelings. The narrative shifts are a happy byproduct.

How do we do this?

First, we bring attention to body sensation. To amplify the sensation and bring the person directly in touch with their body experience, we use movement. Movement in therapy supports embodiment in five ways.

1. Mobilizing or increasing energy in the body. Low-energy clients, whether due to fatigue, depression, or character, benefit from more fully energizing the body. Movement literally requires energy, and it also creates the experience of energy moving through the body.

2. Increasing body awareness. In bioenergetic therapy, asking people to move spontaneously increases their awareness of the somatic experience. In part, this is because the movement of energy in the body generates sensations.

3. Reducing chronic muscular tensions and connective tissue contractions. Movement softens tight muscles in the upper back and neck, as well as the rigidly held shoulders. Softening allows energy—and, therefore, feeling—to flow through those parts. Bioenergetic therapist and massage therapist Lucy Belter reminds me regularly, "Motion is lotion." Loosening chronic constriction requires movement. Helping people to move their constricted parts also helps restore sensation and feeling to those areas.

4. Embodiment of emotional experience. Movement mobilizes energy, which creates sensations. Sensations are the building blocks of feeling awareness in the body. At times, movement generates the flow of emotion very quickly. At other times, it can be a gradual building of somatic experience.

5. Healing and expanding relational capacities. Expressive movement with another person can be reparative. It offers a new and different way of being with one's feelings while relating to another person who is connected and present. This experience can be translated into opportunities for changing relationships in the larger world. It helps an individual explore and develop new ways of relating to other people.

Embodiment is the first step toward expression, which is a step on the path toward processing and integrating. We want people to experience their feelings, contain them without constricting or shutting down, express them appropriately, and let them become part of their self-narrative. By not tying up energy in avoiding feelings, people have access to increased vitality, spontaneity, and clarity. Movement expands the ability to feel and express feelings and is a route for expression not generally available. In therapy, clients actively express themselves through movement. When they have done it in session, it's likely to become part of their home toolkit.

Emotional expression is not the same thing as ungrounded cathartic discharge. We help people gradually experience their own feelings, to integrate parts of the self and connect with reality. Directed movement with reflection builds strong and flexible somatic containers—bodies that are capable of joy, connection, and creativity.

Embodiment and body image

Embodiment is about living your life from your experience of your body. As a practical point, that is the only way that we can live. We are fundamentally somatic beings, but when we have been doing a lot of thinking, we might even feel like disembodied heads floating in space.

Many women live with the idea that their bodies exist for appearance. They think of themselves as the people someone else sees. This objective perspective assumes the body as an object for other people's viewing. When women tell me they "hate" their bodies, they're usually in body-as-object mode. They feel distaste for how they think they appear.

A subjective view is different. Instead of "how does my body look?" the inquiry is "how does my body feel?" Embodiment requires the subjective view. What is it like to be in your body right now? What parts feel good? What parts want your attention? Are there parts that are outside of awareness?

Our focus on sensations in the body requires subjective experiencing of the body. This shifts attention from the belief that how you look is who you are. Embodiment helps women confront conflicts between their subjective experience ("My legs feel strong") and their beliefs about their appearance ("My thighs are fat").

While bioenergetic techniques and activities are not specifically meant to address issues of body image, when we work explicitly with body responses connected to reflection on experiences of embodied living, women shift toward valuing their subjective somatic experience.

Exercise #31: Shaking

Standing in the orienting position, take stock. Check in with yourself, noting breath, body awareness, and any areas of tension. Check into your energy level. Soften your knees and connect your feet to the floor.

Allow your body to shake. You can start with your hands, if you like, then let that motion move up your arms, into your shoulders, and down your torso. Or start with your legs, bouncing your knees up and down. It doesn't matter where you start, just shake. Shake everything you've got to shake and then play around with how you are shaking. Wave your arms overhead, to the side, around your body. Just let it all go. Relax your neck and jaw and make funny noises as your face shakes.

When you begin to tire, allow the movement to slow. Check and see if there is more shaking that your body wants to do.

When you are ready to allow the body to come to stillness, stay with the sensations for a moment. Notice yourself after shaking. What is different? What's the same? How are you aware of energy in your body?

Shaking out is a good exercise if you are overcharged and need to relax and also if you are feeling drowsy and undercharged. It generally relaxes tensions in the body and moves energy around.

Exercise #32: Tighten-Release Exercise to Mobilize Energy

The old-fashioned progressive relaxation exercise is no longer the gold standard for relaxing, but it can be useful in terms of feeling your own energy.

Sitting, lying, or standing, begin with your feet. Tighten your feet and hold. That means squinching up your toes and flexing your soles. Then quickly and consciously, release that tension with a sigh. Now tense your feet and your lower legs. Hold, then release with a gusty sigh.

Now tense your feet, lower legs, thighs, and buttocks (because you can try to separate them, but it isn't easy). Hold for a long moment, then release with a big exhale.

Tense feet, lower legs, thighs, buttocks, your genital area, and your belly. Try to keep your chest, arms, and head soft and relaxed. Hold tightly! Then whoosh, let it all go with a big sigh.

Tense feet, lower legs, thighs, buttocks, genital area, and belly and chest and upper back. Hold while you consciously relax your shoulders, arms and hands, your neck, your face, and scalp. Hold . . . and now whoosh! Let it all go and let go of your breath too.

Tense feet, lower legs, thighs and buttocks, genital area, abdomen, chest, back, shoulders, arms and hands. Squeeze your fists. Tighten everything but keep your neck and face and scalp soft and relaxed. Keep holding and then let everything go. Let out a big sigh and relax.

Finally, tense feet, lower legs, thighs and buttocks, genital area, and abdomen, chest, back, shoulders, arms and hands, your neck, your face, and scalp. Squinch your face all up. Fists, face, toes all as tight as possible. Hold on!

Now whoosh! Let it all go. Let all the tension go. Stand up and shake out your body. Take a moment to check inside. What do you notice now? What has changed?

Exercise #33: Softening the Neck and Jaw

Chronic tensions in the neck and jaw cut off the free flow of emotional energy through the body into the head. We often tense our jaws to keep from saying angry words ("I had to bite my tongue") or to avoid crying. Our necks get tight from keeping the feelings out and from all the mental work we do. It takes energy to keep those muscles chronically tense. Softening the neck and jaw can open up more feeling.

Standing in the orienting position, knees soft and feet firmly grounded, let your head settle on your neck. Take a moment to notice any sensations that are present. Now very slowly and gently, tilt your head to the side so that your ear is approaching your shoulder. Let your shoulder stay where it is, but gently invite the ear to come closer. Then allow your head to lift back to center, and now allow the other ear to approach the relevant shoulder. Slow is key!

Return to center and slowly drop your chin toward your chest. Breathe here, then lift your chin again and turn your head to the side. Let your eyes lead the way, but keep your body oriented forward.

Only your neck and head turn. Be gentle. There is no prize for turning farther. Then slowly return to center and repeat on the other side.

You can repeat the whole sequence, even adding some easy neck rolls from side to side if that feels good. If you like, you can use your hands to massage the back of your neck or wherever you feel tightness.

When you decide to finish, take a moment standing on your feet and check in again. What did you get from that?

Are you more aware of your body messages after you have completed this sequence? You might notice some overall relaxation along with changes in your breathing.

CHAPTER 13

Emotions in Therapy: Anger

Many people experience their emotional lives as confusing, chaotic, and unmanageable. Afraid of their feelings, as if a wave of body sensation could harm them or others, they constrict and repress, explode and collapse, suffering instead of living.

Therapy creates a welcoming space for emotion. Somatic therapists bring permission to emotional expression, setting limits only when necessary for safety. There is a wide range of available expression that doesn't breach those limits.

We may not realize it, but there are social constraints on the expression of all emotions, including joy, pleasure, and happiness. We don't condone full body expression of these feelings, at least not in adults and often not in children. It is almost as if feelings are supposed to be private, only discussed but never experienced in the company of others. Therapy changes all of that.

Our clients may be "happy," but they probably haven't jumped for joy, or danced around with euphoria, or screamed with terror, despite feeling those emotions. They may not cry with despair, hit or kick with anger, or collapse into grief. In fact, most of my clients are actively involved in preventing somatic expressions of their bodies' deep feelings.

Bodies have movements to go with emotions, and we are taught from an early age to suppress them. We teach children not to hit (of course) or scream or jump around. These behaviors complicate things and can even hurt other people. However, the message that children learn is that there is something wrong with the feelings themselves.

Somatic therapists support people to find their authentic movements that express their feelings. Using those movements allows the feeling to be "completed" in the body. This practice processes emotions authentically, contributing to integration of the self.

Emotional granularity

Having a rich vocabulary of emotion helps people to experience their emotions more completely. Think about your own experiences of anger. Can you recall times when you were angry about different things, or with different people? Did you notice any differences in how you experienced those feelings? We tend to differentiate anger from frustration and rage, but in some cultures there are words for many more finely graded variations on anger. What are some of the categories of anger you have experienced or can imagine experiencing?

Becoming aware of the fine distinctions within and between emotion categories in your own experience makes it possible for you to feel more. To make the distinction, you must attend deeply to your experience, and that attention gives you a richer emotional experience. But to even start, you cannot be afraid of your feelings. In therapy, you help clients to tolerate and ultimately befriend emotion, increasing capacity for self-possession.

Exercises for emotional expression

Anger distresses perinatal clients, partly due to unrealistic images of motherhood. They are modeling themselves after an ideal, and the anger, frustration, and even rage they feel isn't part of that model. Anger is an everyday part of parenting, though, so there is value in becoming acquainted.

Exploring emotion in a contained way is often very helpful. Working with expression brings up whatever is present. You might think you're working with anger but feel sadness or fear. Many women cry while expressing anger, for example. They report feeling a confusing mixture, perhaps because our culture does not support women's anger. Expressing whatever arises will often unpack layers of feelings, leading to more openness and clarity.

Practicing the exercises below supports you in flowing with the wave of feeling as it arises and recedes. Since anger often covers fear, sadness, or despair, don't be surprised at all the feelings that might come up. Stay with your compassionate curiosity and see what you can learn about yourself. Once you have become comfortable doing this work yourself, you can explore it with your clients.

Working with the energy of anger

We are so used to wearing our social masks that our facial expressions often don't match our feelings. A simple practice of allowing the feeling to show its face can be helpful to both emotional granularity and to decreasing emotional distress.

Exercise #34: Take Down the Mask

This exercise came from a bioenergetic training workshop with Michael Maley, PhD.

Think about the masks we wear daily. We are so accustomed to our masked selves that we may not even realize we are wearing masks. I have clients who smile reflexively, even when recounting the most horrific life experiences. They are often unaware of how they look and sometimes unaware of how they feel.

Place your hand across the top of your forehead and slide it down over your face, imagining that you are sliding off your mask. Go very slowly so that you can ease that mask right off. Then let your face assume the look of how you are feeling. If that is too hard, just take a look at your face without your mask. How does it look? What do you think that person is feeling inside?

Now think about playing with the mask of anger. Can you narrow your eyes? Stick out your lower jaw? What about sticking out your tongue or making a really mean face? Bare your teeth. Is there a sound? If you can feel a growl or a hiss inside, let it come out. Glare at the mirror or just at the wall. Let your face show anger.

Now draw down that mask. Let your face rest in neutral again. How does it feel to wear an angry face? A neutral face? What is your usual face?

Since the pandemic of 2020, we've had to deal with actual face masks, but we've dealt with social masks for many years before that. Notice what it is like inside you when you wear your social mask and when you allow your face to express your internal reality.

Exercise #35: Expression with a Hand Towel

Start in the orienting position, either standing or sitting. Press your feet into the floor and feel the contours of your body. Take note of where you are in space. Take a breath and feel the changes in your body as you inhale and exhale. This is the container.

Now grasp a hand towel with both hands. Try twisting it in your lap. Now lift it up to eye level and twist the towel. Narrow your eyes and stick out your lower jaw. Twist hard.

Watch your inner experience. What is happening inside you as you twist and narrow and stick out your jaw?

Drop the towel and take a deep breath. What has changed in you?

Now think of an annoying or irritating circumstance. You can even think of something that made you angry, if it is easy to access. Press your feet into the floor and then lift the towel again. How can you express the feeling using the towel? Narrow your eyes, jut your jaw, and twist, shake, snap, do whatever you want with that towel to express how your body is feeling right now. If there is a sound your body wants to make, let it come out. Let the movement and sound continue while you feel the flow of energy through you. Follow your body's desire to keep twisting, hitting, shaking, or what have you. When the impulse to move eases away, let the movement slow to a close. Take a moment to press your feet, feel your breath, and notice what changed in you because of the exercise.

Some people find an immediate resistance to expressing anger. I have had clients stop entirely to tell me that they are not angry, or that they don't like anger, or that they don't want to be angry. I encourage them to continue, because they don't have to be angry to do this exercise.

It is, after all, just an exercise. If they are not already angry, playing with a towel isn't going to make them get angry.

If, however, they are afraid that something as minor as playing with a towel will unleash something terrifying, then they need to do this exercise to see that they do, in fact, have control. The truism we state in therapy is that feeling isn't the same as doing, but for many people that makes no sense at all. They are afraid of feeling because they don't think they will be able to control their behavior when they feel what they feel. Exercises like this one create an experience in which a person titrates their own contact with emotion and controls how and when she touches it. Feel, kiss, flow.

Exercise #36: Expressing Anger by Pushing

Start in the orienting position, feet pressing into the floor. Take a few breaths to feel the container of your body. Note your current state.

You're going to be pushing against something for this exercise. You can use the wall, the big exercise ball pressed against the wall, or a tall piece of furniture. Find the place where you will push and offset your feet so that you can push from your core—the center of your belly—without losing your footing. That is, put one foot about twelve inches ahead of the other so you'll be able to lean safely into pushing. Then push against the surface with straight arms. It is best if there is a little give but no danger of the surface giving way. We're just working with expression through the arms.

Narrow your eyes and stick out your jaw. Push, push, push. Get a rhythm going where you push a few times, then ease back and take stock. How are you feeling doing this pushing? What images, thoughts, feelings, and sensations arise in you as you push and back away? Are there words or sounds that come up? What is it like in your body when you let the sounds accompany the movement?

Exercise #37: Variation: Pushing with Another Person

If you are pushing with another person, ask them to give you return pressure but only enough to keep contact. In this case, you'll push enough to feel that you are pushing but don't try to push them over. Monitor the flow of your energy and feeling as you push, push, push, and release. Notice the flow of energy between you. Is there a struggle for power happening? How do you experience this?

Try pushing with eye contact. Now try pushing without looking at their eyes. What is each of these like? Notice how you feel about the other person as you do this. Does he or she take on a different appearance as your feelings rise and subside?

❧

I keep a variety of throw pillows in the office because they are eminently useful. One thing they're useful for is, yes, throwing.

I can toss a client a pillow and watch how she handles it. Sometimes she'll grab it to her midsection and use it for protection and comfort. Sometimes she'll shake it a bit or squeeze it. If it looks like moving the pillow might move some emotion, I invite her to throw it across the room against the wall. Most people find this fun and amusing. If it seems productive, I invite her to stand and throw pillow after pillow at the wall, while I gather them up and hand them over, one at a time. I watch and invite a grounded stance and a two-handed throw over the head, which is likely to move the most energy. If she tries that but prefers another stance, I watch and listen. This exercise seems to be enlivening and not very threatening at all, perhaps because of the playfulness. Again, try it yourself several times before offering it to a client.

Exercise #38: Throwing Pillows

Gather a pile of pillows on one side of your room. Clear the wall on the other side, being especially mindful that throws can easily go wide. Hold a pillow by the corners well over your head and fling it hard at the opposite wall. Keep your feet grounded, knees soft, and throw hard. See the best place to stand to get a satisfying thwack against the far wall. Then gather up your pillows and do another round.

As you gather momentum, see if there is a sound you can let out when you release the pillow. There might also be words. Let the words come and notice how that changes your experience.

When you feel the impulse slow, take a break to settle into the orienting position, feeling your feet press the ground and your breath moving. Take a few breaths to see what you got from this experience. Stay open to whatever arises.

Rage: A special case

Rage isn't just anger, it's a powerful distillation of unmet needs that tends to erupt rather than be experienced. When a woman tells me about her rage, I wonder what she's not getting that she desperately needs. Just as toddlers will rage when their needs are not met, so will parents. When there is rage, it is an emotional emergency. Unfortunately, we tend to treat it as a behavioral disaster.

Let's look more deeply. Other people's rage is frightening because a raging person deploys any available weapons—screaming, saying mean things, and sometimes even physical violence. These are forms of energetic discharge that are damaging both to the person who receives and to the person who is raging. Our own rage is frightening because of the feeling of being out of control of oneself. Nobody likes it. Toddlers who have regular raging meltdowns are not doing it because they like it. They are doing it because they desperately need something, and they don't know how to get it.

Parents are exactly the same. Rage erupts when we are desperate—for a moment of quiet, for control over the situation, for a bit of connection from our loved one, or even for sleep or food. We can't tell what we need in the moment, so we tend to frame it as a projection. That is, mothers will tell me that they need their children to do what they are told or their spouse to help clean up and stop playing on his phone.

The underlying need is probably something else, perhaps a need to feel in control of her own life or a need to feel cared for.

Parents who rage often don't recognize their own gradual ramping up of reactivity. They may deny anger and perhaps genuinely struggle to feel it. When we work with anger in therapy, we help people to recognize the body cues that tell them they are getting overcharged. Learning to experience your own anger in a manageable way means that you don't have to suppress it until it boils over.

Mothers tell me that they are "doing good" with the kids, but that the kids just keep on pushing their buttons. The "doing good" means that the parent is actively suppressing her annoyance, frustration, and irritation to meet some idealized standard of motherhood, not that she is genuinely tolerating the demands of being with the children. She's hiding her response, even from herself.

Keeping the kids happy isn't a reasonable parenting goal, especially with toddlers.

Keeping them safe, helping them learn, and modeling clear boundaries and self-respect are reasonable goals. Those goals mean that kids are going to be unhappy at times. For example, nobody wants to stop playing when it is time to leave. If a mother judges her parenting by how happy her children are, and many do, she may prioritize their momentary satisfaction over her own needs. She may not notice the insistent small voice inside her that is the steam rising from an incipient volcano. Parents tell me that they explode without warning, but it is often because they are not attuned to their own warning signals.

Doing the work on anger (including frustration, irritation, annoyance, and edginess) will help clients to take that break, shift energetic gears, and come back to ground before rage takes over.

CHAPTER 14

Emotions in Therapy: Sadness and Joy

Sadness and grief are an inevitable part of life. While sadness is an emotion, grief is an entire somatic experience. Grieving takes over a person's sleep, appetite, digestion, and energy processes. In the early days of a loss, the grieving process is continuous, but over time grieving becomes more intermittent. Waves of grief wash over the bereaved, usually unexpectedly, often accompanied by strong expressions of sadness, longing, and despair. Bereaved people often understand that grieving is a process, and they need space and time to grieve. However, in our hurry culture, people are expected to "get on with it" much sooner than bodies are ready to complete grieving.

In our practice, it is helpful to make space for grief, even without bereavement. There are losses that accompany any birth, including the loss of a woman's autonomy, her prior identity, her identity as a pregnant person, and her idealized images of both her baby and herself as a mother. This grieving process can be complicated by beliefs that she "should" be happy with her baby and that she has nothing to be mad or sad about.

We encourage her to use movement to express whatever she is feeling. By watching her small spontaneous movements, we can often infer an emotional process and invite her to expand on it. A clenched fist, a sagging jaw, upwelling tears all hint at feelings that can be invited in.

Grief is a weight bearing down on us. We can help support her body through this weighty process. Offer her space to lie down. Support her feet with pillows. Offer a cuddly blanket. Encourage her to seek out somatic comfort measures to support her body with processing her grief.

Sadness often brings tears and great sobs that originate in the lower abdomen. Clients often reflexively suppress their crying, even in your office. Notice how they might be cutting off the feeling and expression. You can see tensing of the neck and jaw, looking away, trying to change the subject. They won't assume that you are okay with their tears unless you show them by inviting them to let the feeling come up.

You can also help clients who want to cry by inviting sobbing through movement and using the voice. They can vocalize by sighing as they exhale, then adding volume to the sigh. If you sigh along with them, they often feel freer to make noise. Open-mouth vocalizing, or sounding, opens channels that can release sobbing.

Exercise #39: Using Breath to Invite Sobbing

As always, directions are written for you to practice before offering the exercise to your clients.

From the orienting position, allow your head to lead you down into the forward bend, arms dangling from the shoulders. Sigh deeply as you let your legs support you, knees soft, and your upper body just relaxes by hanging over. Let your neck go and wiggle your jaw to be sure you are not holding it.

Eyes open, allow a long sound to come out of your open mouth as you exhale. You'll be looking at your knees or the wall behind you. Inhale and then let out another long sound. Listen to the sound of your voice.

Now deepen the bend in your soft knees, then straighten them while pressing your feet into the floor and pushing your lower back toward the ceiling. Repeat. This time, exhale when you push, making a sound. Continue to bend and straighten your legs, sounding on the exhalation as you press your lower back toward the ceiling. Let your exhalations and sounds be long.

With the next exhalation, breathe out until you cannot breathe out anymore, then push a little, and a little more. Make a sobbing sound with your breath at the end of your exhalation, then allow the spontaneous inhalation. Repeat. Notice if your body wants to take this over. If you feel sobbing begin, allow it to happen. Often sobs will feel like they are coming from low in the belly, rippling up and out while you are in the bent-over position. Notice if you can open this channel to whatever arises. Allow your body to process whatever is coming up.

Sobbing, with or without tears, may continue for a few minutes and the discharge of energy will naturally wind down to an end. You can also end it anytime you wish by resting your hands on your thighs, then slowly pushing your hands into your thighs as you rise upright. Stand solidly on your two feet. Notice your connection to the ground. If you feel disoriented, bend and straighten your knees, pushing your feet into the floor. When you feel grounded, take a deep breath or a few and look around the room. Do you notice anything different?

Exercise #40: Opening the Chest

Any movement that expands the chest, and therefore the breathing, may open a channel to the diaphragm for sobbing. Here are three simple ways to open the chest.

A. In a standing position, spread your arms out wide, then bend your elbows and put your hands behind your head. Notice your heart, right there in the middle of your chest. Lift your heart, just a bit, by pulling your elbows together slightly. What do you notice? Now see if you can let out a long breath, like the candle-blowing breath mentioned earlier. When you inhale, notice where your breath goes. Repeat. Exhale again with a big sigh. Drop your jaw and let the sound come out. Notice the sound. What do you hear in your sigh?

B. Lie backward over a yoga ball, feet firmly planted on the floor. If your neck is very tight, shape a hand towel into a small roll to support your neck. Bring your arms back and over your head, feet still firmly on the floor. Move around on the ball and feel your body connecting. Then with your arms back or behind your head, exhale as above, a long breath with a sigh. Repeat. Notice your awareness of the expansion of your chest, the lifting of your heart, and the sound of your sigh.

C. In the previous exercise, the curvature of the ball helped to open the chest. You can get a similar effect while lying on a flat surface by using a roll under the chest. Use a bath towel rolled tightly or a foam roller under the back while lying on the floor. Place the roll horizontal to the body at mid chest. If your neck is too tight to be here comfortably, use a hand towel to create a little lift for your head. We do want a small stretch here. Rest arms comfortably at your side or stretched along the floor above your head. Breathe as directed above. Focus on the exhale with a sigh as you notice the expansion and opening in your chest. Notice whatever arises as you continue to sigh out the air.

Often, this kind of expansion plus the breathing plus the gentle, low-pressure vocalization will bring up sadness. If the diaphragm can release a bit here, the body may sob. A few moments may be enough in any of these positions.

Follow up with a forward bend (Exercise #13) to help your client ground. Be aware that emotion may begin to flow during the grounding, so encourage your client to rest into the forward bend and just feel whatever she feels. There will be time to talk about it later.

Working with the energies of joy, pleasure, and satisfaction

Joy, pleasure, and satisfaction are all on the continuum of happiness, but they can feel different from each other and can be expressed in different ways. People are more likely to have some granularity of the experiences of "happiness" than anger or sadness, but they may not have many channels for somatic expression.

Many mindfulness practices focus on sensory awareness. Bioenergetics goes further to invite attention to sensory pleasure. I use these kinds of exercises repeatedly with clients who are presenting with depression. One of the most debilitating parts of depressive disorders that people experience is the lack of interest and lack of pleasure. I invite them to seek out pleasurable experiences just to remind themselves that they have the capacity to enjoy. It can be very hard to access that capacity when the fog of depression is thick.

Try these exercises yourself, of course.

Exercise #41: Sensory Channels

Think about what you especially enjoy. What brings you a gentle sense of pleasure in your body? It can be the feeling of a hot mug of tea in your hand, the texture of a cuddly blanket, the fur of your pet. Or maybe it is the smell of baking bread, roses, or your lavender essential oil. Perhaps your pleasure comes from the melting sweetness of chocolate on your tongue, the crisp crunch of a fall apple. You might be more auditory and get the most pleasure from birdsong or whispers from your child. Which sensory pathway is most sensitive to pleasure?

During the day, indulge that sensory pleasure. It only takes a moment to savor the warmth of your mug in your hand, but if you don't take that moment, you might miss the pleasure. When you pick up your mug, take the time to notice exactly what is so enjoyable to you. Let the experience sink down deep into you. Allow yourself to savor the pleasure of the moment.

When people have depression, the sensations may be unavailable to them. Inviting them to notice where they once found pleasure can be a painful reminder of how low they feel. However, checking to see if there is anything at all that they can appreciate about the moment can help orient them toward finding pleasure.

If you happen to notice your client enjoying something in your office, you can check in. "Do you like that blanket? It's nice to see you enjoying it." It is not a big deal, but you help her to notice that yes, there is something that is a little enjoyable. Bring your curiosity to her experience. Help her to be a detective about what she likes and what helps her feel good.

Exercise #42: Expression of Joy

Sometimes you are a witness to your clients' joys. People will tell you how they want to express their joy, but they may not allow themselves the full expression. "I wanted to jump with joy!" could be read as an invitation to a somatic therapist. Such a movement, like many others in somatic therapies, is best accomplished together. Invite her up to her feet to do it with you. Jumping around like a little kid is an experience you don't allow yourself as an adult. Demonstrate your pleasure in your client's joy.

You can also use your mirroring and attunement skills to support the expression of joy. Perhaps jumping for joy isn't feasible in your office, but you could mirror her joyful expression and attune with the affect (emotional expression) and the idea with excited clapping or bouncing in your chair. This increases your alliance with her and helps her feel her joy more acutely.

If you have space and time, Exercise #23: The Joy of Being Alive in Chapter 10 could be a good addition.

Exercise #43: Relief and Satisfaction (How Much Is Enough?)

Many mothers struggle to find satisfaction in their lives. Instead, there's a feeling of never being enough or never having enough. This complex issue can be alleviated by heightening an awareness of satisfaction when it occurs, and even more simply, noticing relief.

When you are doing something that challenges you and you stop, there is often a sense of relief. Try this. Stand with your weight on both feet. Now shift to the right so you are putting most of your weight on your right leg and foot, using your left toes for balance only. Bend and straighten your right knee, moving very slowly. Keep going. It won't take long for your right leg to begin to tire; notice that and feel the protest in your muscles. Keep bending and straightening until you are strongly aware of a desire to stop this movement. Take that strong awareness and say, "That's enough!" loudly as you return to two feet.

Notice how it feels. What is relief like in your leg? In the rest of your body? What was it like to protest and then feel relief?

Is there any satisfaction there?

Satisfaction can exist without relief too. Satisfaction arises in the completion of a movement. It is a body state that arises at the end of a trajectory. After doing the throwing pillows exercise, for example, you may experience a sense of satisfaction.

Satisfaction can arise without your noticing, but increasing your awareness of satisfying activities supports a sense of a satisfying life. You can notice satisfaction around eating. If you are aware of your hunger, your desire for a particular food, and the process of meeting that need and want, you may also be able to notice when that need/want has been satisfied. What does satisfaction feel like in this context? Look for satisfaction in other activities too. If you are exercising, when does your body feel satisfied that you have done enough?

When you are having a conversation, does it end with a sense of satisfaction? Or do you feel "loose ends" that are not complete? How does it feel in your body to have an unsatisfying interaction? The idea of satisfaction as somatic may be foreign at first, but there are distinct body sensations associated with your sense that something has been completed to your, well, satisfaction.

Learn to notice what feels satisfying to you and your body's sense of satisfaction. Encourage your clients to do the same.

Overwhelm

Many new mothers report feeling overwhelmed by the expectations, tasks, and emotional load of new parenting. Getting some of that load off the back of the client can free her up to function better. Tolerating overwhelm is an essential skill.

Try this exercise yourself before doing it with clients.

Exercise #44: Working with Overwhelm/Get Off My Back

Standing in the orienting position, press your feet into the floor, feeling your body in the space and allowing your breath to flow.

Think about the load you carry. Your work, your family, your responsibilities. Is there anything you might like to unload? Keeping your feet planted and your hips facing forward, bend one arm and thrust your elbow back. Make the same movement with your other arm. Try it a few more times.

Now narrow your eyes, stick out your jaw, and thrust one elbow back. Try some words, such as "Get off my back!" You can let your head turn along with your elbow or just keep facing forward. Try both ways and see what effect that has on your experience.

You can also try both elbows at the same time, noticing how your body responds to that.

When you've expressed this for a while, take a moment to shake out and see what you notice. Does your body want to do this exercise again? If yes, do it again and see how it changes.

In bringing this exercise to a client, do it along with her. You are modeling the movement and encouraging her vocalization. Make time and space for her to settle and reflect on her experience. She may notice a sense of satisfaction after getting some things off her back.

Exercise #45: Throwing Off Our Burdens

The feeling of overwhelm is unpleasant. Another way to lighten the load of overwhelm is a throwing exercise in which you invite the client to pitch her worries or burdens away from her, perhaps out the window of your therapy room. These imagined burdens won't break your window.

As usual, practice this on your own first.

Stand in the orienting position, considering the many things that you have on your back. Taking a staggered stance, imagine that you are throwing a burden off your back and away from you. Reach your arms back over your head, grab an imaginary something, and throw it over your head and out the window or into the pile in the middle of the room.

Keep throwing and piling up those nasty burdens. Narrow your eyes, stick out your jaw, and tell them to "get off my back!" or whatever words arise for you.

Throw until your body tells you to take a break. Your body knows when you've had enough. Then return to the orienting position, check your grounding, and breathe.

What did you get from that? How does your body feel now? Can you feel a shift?

As above, do this exercise with your client. If she gets into it with enthusiasm, you can take the role of cheerleader as well as model.

☙ CHAPTER 15 ☙

Mother-Infant Interventions

Being a mother means different things to different women, and the concept of "being a mother" and the actual practice of it may not be aligned. That is, if you ask a woman about mothering, she will tell you what she thinks. If you are with her while she is interacting with her baby, you will be able to observe how her ideas of herself as mother play out. If you are very lucky, you'll catch your clients on bad days as well as good days so that you can grasp the breadth of their experiences. Of course, there are limits to what you can observe: no therapist that I know goes home with mothers to spend long wakeful nights trying to get the baby to sleep.

Exercise #46: Shower of Affirmation

Some of what happens when a mother and baby are together in your office, or during home visits, will inform you about how the mechanics of the relationship are working. Does the pair seem to dance comfortably together? Are there places where they seem to be well-synchronized, understanding each other's signals and moving from connection to disconnection and back to connection with minimal distress?

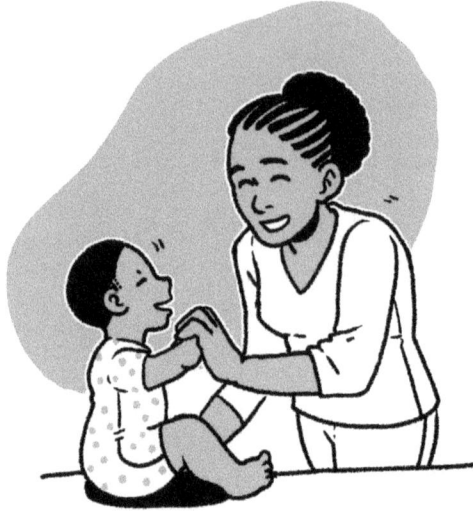

These are moments to be identified and lauded. Mothers often do very well on their own, without even realizing it. Like all of us, they tend to pay more attention to the places that don't feel good, where there is an identifiable struggle. But first and always, it helps to look for what is going well and what is right about the two of them together.

Use your body resonance to feel into the relationship as you sit with mother and infant. Notice and comment positively on connection, on the baby's developmental shifts, and the mother's ease. Studiously avoid offering a critique. This is a shower of affirmation of the dyad in front of you. Ask her what she's noticing or even what she likes best about their interactions. With some dyads, it can be very hard to see the dance because the pair is out of synchronicity. Your goal is to reflect material that support her sense of competency in mothering. You can use your mirroring and attunement practices here as well as with the mother.

The baby is a potent releaser of all sorts of psychological responses, thoughts, feelings, beliefs, projections, memories, and fantasies. It is helpful to ask the mother what she notices in herself as she is attending to the baby. Watch her look at the baby and then gently ask, "What do you notice inside yourself as you look at him?" Watch her body response to the baby and to your inquiry. Remember that at this point in her life her attention is extremely oriented to this baby. She may be completely unaware of what the child brings up in her, but that is what is driving her thoughts, feelings, and behavior. Listen hard to what she tells you. Keep noticing your own body responses.

If she reports on processes of thinking, ask her to check in with her body, specifically her chest and belly, to see what she notices there as she gazes at her baby. This supports her dual awareness in which she is aware of the baby and how the interaction affects her internal state.

Case Example #4: Anique's baby reminds her of her abusive ex

Anique is a first-time parent, twenty-five, and Samuel is three months old. Anique separated from her husband due to physical and emotional abuse just a month before the baby's birth.

"He looks so much like my husband," states Anique. "Sometimes he looks at me like he hates me. I think he might hate me for leaving his father. He's going to have a single mother, and it is my fault."

This is an opportunity to work directly with the mother-baby relationship, and she's provided a strong feeling word, suggesting access to somatic experience. I engage my compassionate curiosity, wondering how she feels when she thinks her baby hates her. Does she confuse her baby with his father? What is she feeling?

"That must be hard. Is he doing it now?"

"No, not now. Usually, it is only when he is crying. He glares at me and I . . ." She chokes up and stops speaking.

"When he cries sometimes it feels like he's mad at you," I encourage. "What is that like?"

She glares at me. "Terrible, what do you think? To have your little baby mad at you. That feels terrible."

I am nothing if not persistent. "Yeah, I bet it does feel terrible. Like sick to your stomach? Or scary? Or something else?"

She ponders, then responds. "Yeah, mostly like, why do I try? He's going to hate me just like his father does, and why do I even think I can do this? I feel tired and beaten down when that happens."

I am aware of my desire to reassure her or tell her that she won't always feel that way. I also don't think that's what she needs, even though it might meet my need. I am uncomfortable with her struggle, but I can tolerate my own discomfort. Instead, I try to make space for whatever she needs to say.

"I bet that does feel pretty awful, and then you have a crying baby who needs you too."

"Yep. It is hard to do what I have to do." We take a moment of silence to hear that. She is doing what she must do, and we both know that it is hard.

I bring her back to the here and now. "Right now, looking at him, what do you notice?"

She gazes down at the baby in her arms. "He's pretty cute. His hair, he's losing his hair. The new hair is lighter. And I think his eyes look like my mother, actually." She looks up with a smile.

"And what do you notice inside you as you talk about him?"

"I feel pretty good. He's had a good day, and so I feel like maybe we can do this."

I match her smile and nod. "This is a good moment. We all need good moments to put in our pockets to remember when things are hard."

She laughed. "Like having a piece of candy in your pocket."

"Right. Let's notice what makes this moment feel pretty good." I invite her to describe her comfort on the couch, how she feels while holding her sleeping baby, and her warm-hearted feelings for him. Giving attention to this shift allows her to expand her thinking.

"When I see him like this, I remember that he is only a little dude, and he really doesn't know anything to be mad about."

I nod my encouragement. "He is only a little dude."

"Yeah, and most of the time we do pretty good."

"And sometimes he has hard days. Because babies have hard days."

"Yes. We both do."

"Yeah, of course. He's new at being a person and you're new at being his mom." We breathe and look at the baby while she allows that idea to penetrate. After I moment, I offer, "When he's crying a lot, I wonder if it might be a reminder or like a trigger to bring up old stuff from your marriage?"

"Oh, yeah. When I'm so tired I could die, I'm furious that I have to do this alone. I don't want my ex back, but I don't want to have to be a single parent. He's the bad one, and he sleeps at night."

"Unfair."

"So unfair. It makes me so mad." Her face reflects that feeling.

"I'm sure you do get furious. And exhausted."

"I don't want to be furious. I want to be a good mom to Samuel and forget about all that bad stuff. But I feel so defeated when the baby keeps on crying."

"Is that a reminder?"

She thinks. "Yeah, feeling defeated. I always felt like I couldn't do anything right. No matter what I did, my ex was mad about it, or mad at me, or something. He was loud too. Loud meant bad things were going to happen."

"So when Samuel gets loud . . ."

"Yeah, maybe. Maybe I get scared. And then I guess maybe I think it is the baby's fault. He's mad at me and scaring me." There is a pause. "But he's really just a baby, right?"

"He's just a baby."

"When I get upset it's easy for me to forget that. Think he hates me. But he doesn't. He's just upset, too."

"That makes sense." We think about that together for a moment.

She gazes into the baby's face. "Such a sweet boy," she murmurs. "I just wish I could feel this when he's screaming."

In that moment she puts into words what so many wish for, a magic way to keep your cool when the baby is losing his. "How does it go when he's crying?"

"Depends. If he's hungry and I feed him, then that's fine. It's when I can't figure out why he's crying and he gets so upset, that's when I lose it too."

"When you lose it, what happens?"

"It's like my head is spinning, like I can't think. He glares at me, I feel worse and worse, and I want to put him down but he screams harder and I just can't stand it."

Her head spins and she "can't stand it." I grimace, mirroring the face she's making. "Are you feeling any of that now?"

"Not really, but my stomach gets a little tense telling you about it. I lose my sense of him as a baby and me as the adult when he won't stop crying. I wish I could get some perspective, but how do I do that when I am already upset?"

"It's hard when you feel your head spinning and like your feet won't hold you," I agree. "Right here, while you're feeling okay, let's practice a couple of things that might help."

While she sits, holding the sleeping baby, she pushes her feet into the floor and her body into the couch. Grounding through feeling the contours of her body and pressing her feet into the floor helps with that disembodied feeling. She agrees that she could try that strategy when she feels her head spinning.

With support, she also generates some phrases to use as re-minders when agitated. I write them down for her. We also talk about using earplugs to soften the loudness of the baby's cries so that she can respond to him without reacting in fear.

Countertransference

Countertransference is when the therapist projects beliefs or expecta-tions onto the client. It is quite normal and needs our awareness to keep it from derailing the therapy. After all, therapy is about the client, not the therapist.

There are times when we treat a client differently than others and it is not due to countertransference. We must follow up if we assess her as suicidal, of course, or hear that there is danger to her or the baby in the home. Therapists likely have strong feelings about those issues, but they are not necessarily caused by countertransference. However, working with mothers and infants is enormously evocative. At times, our thoughts or feelings about the mother are reflections of our own history. When we react to a client from our personal history, that's countertransference in action.

Countertransference shows up in different ways. A therapist might feel stressed by a particular client, or angry at how she's being treated, or angry at her for how she's treating her baby. Sometimes we want to rescue her from her life or rescue the baby from the mother. Strong attraction, repulsion, irritation, or annoyance with a client are signals. We are attributing something to this client that likely is from our own history, even if we can't figure it out.

Keeping an awareness of ourselves while being with the mother in her struggle is critically important. When a client's struggles are similar to those we've experienced, we may expect her to react as we did, or we may find ourselves reactive when she does something different. If we are facing our worst fears in the form of our client's life, that might bleed into the session. It is our work to develop and maintain awareness of our own tender spots, so we recognize when we are activated. Then we take steps to contain ourselves.

It's okay when client work brings up your own struggle. You bracket it for later; it doesn't belong in her session, but you'll have it for your own work. Right now, everything is about the client in front of you.

When you become aware you have been activated this way, congratulate yourself! You have caught the countertransference. Now you can decide what to do about it. Look at how you think and feel about this client compared to others. How has that affected your interactions? Can you limit the effect? This is what I mean by "bracketing" the countertransference. Infant distress distresses everyone, so when the baby fusses or even gets extremely upset, you have an opportunity. It's a wonderful chance to help your client check in with herself. It is also likely to generate some countertransferential "stuff" for you.

What comes up for your client when the fussing starts? What comes up in your mind as the therapist/support person? Asking the client may need to wait until she has calmed the baby.

Stay in your dual awareness as you watch her comfort him. Notice what she does, how she responds, and how your own body responds to what is going on.

Is she able to give him a little space and time to self-soothe or does she leap immediately to full-on comfort measures?

Does she start with her voice and eyes before going straight to picking him up? What is her level of reactivity to his distress? Overall, can you assess her tolerance for fussing or crying? Later you may want to explore what she is saying to herself about her mothering.

As an intervention, note and remark on all that's going well. "He's really good at letting you know he wants something," is a useful comment, particularly when her inner critic is telling her that he's crying because she's a terrible mother.

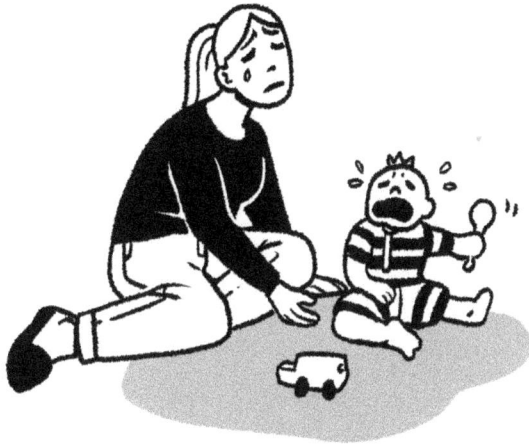

Crying babies and countertransference

Are you able to separate your beliefs about mothering/parenting from hers? Notice particularly if there is a part of you that wants to intervene and what your internal voice is saying.

It can sometimes be challenging to be another adult in the room when a baby is fussing and the mother is struggling. Therapists can feel strong urges to "help out" by taking the baby or by offering advice on baby handling. Beware! Your client probably has a mother and in-laws who perhaps already do this, and she likely has a formidable pile of mixed feelings about it. You are not here to help her parent, at least not directly. Keeping your role very clear is necessary (and often difficult).

It is essential to keep in mind that the woman is your client and your job is to help her become an autonomous and comfortable mother. Make your decisions about what to do and when to do it based on your theoretical framework, which tells you how people develop and learn. That way, you will probably make good decisions.

It is rarely helpful to "rescue" the baby from the mother as that is likely to reinforce her own sense of incompetence. On occasion, you may need to hold the baby while the mother takes a moment to breathe, perhaps with a washroom break, but if the baby is still crying when she returns that's probably a good thing. It would be unfortunate for you to be more "successful" in the moment than the mother. She is already depending on you for a lot, and part of that dependency is your "knowing" that she is capable of being a competent mother to her baby and, in fact, the best mother for her baby.

"Rescue" fantasies are not uncommon in therapists who work with challenged parents. They are best understood as countertransferential and a reflection of the therapist's deep desire to be helpful, though "rescue" is not your mode of helping. Like other forms of countertransference, it's useful to bracket the experience.

Sometimes tucking the information into the bracket is sufficient, but if a mother stirs you, discussing the countertransference in supervision is an excellent way to get support. If you've uncovered something deeply challenging, taking it to your own therapist is a great idea. Perinatal clients bring up a lot in all of us, and getting support while you are working in this field is a great investment in yourself.

Case Example #5: Karen is a competent mom

Karen's baby, Darcy, age six months, is with her in the office. Her toddler is home with Grandma.

Darcy is inconsolable, perhaps needing sleep as her mom is preparing to leave at the end of her appointment. Karen has to use the washroom before leaving and hands Darcy to me to hold.

Darcy continues to register his extreme distress. I try to "be with" Darcy, reminding him that his mother will be right back, trying to channel my inner Kent Hoffman from Circle of Security. Darcy is having none of it, and when Karen returns, he continues to cry. I state the obvious: "He is not happy."

Karen grins happily at me. I am aware that my allegiance with her is strengthened by the fact that Darcy would not settle for me either.

"He'll be okay," she says confidently. "He'll go to sleep in the car."

I grin. "You're the mom."

Beyond helping the mother to become reflective about her inner process as she is interacting with her baby, there are specific ways you can modify bioenergetic activities to include this important dyad.

Helping the baby to relax the body using the mother's breathing

Within the realm of perinatal treatment, mothers can learn to use their breath to help their babies soften and relax. A mother who can't be bothered to help herself feel better will nevertheless use all sorts of things to try to help her baby.

Case Example #6: Maria's baby worries her

Maria, ten days postpartum, has come to the prenatal and pediatric clinic where I supervise our case management program. Marie is very upset. Levi has been vomiting every time he eats, as well as between feedings, and he cries continually. Sleep has been almost non-existent. Maria's husband is supportive but is at work most of the time.

Maria is beside herself. She has no idea what is happening, and she is terribly afraid that she is somehow killing her baby. She knows that babies spit up, but she did not expect it from her baby—at least not to such an extreme.

While our nurse practitioner contacts our on-call pediatrician, I sit with Maria and Levi.

Previously, I had been present for an episode of vomiting that helped me to understand we are dealing with something atypical. No wonder Maria is frightened. Both she and the baby are tense, disconnected, and suffering.

Maria and I know each other from her prenatal visits. In our mother-baby room, she sits in the rocker holding Levi, who cries inconsolably. I sit with them and watch and listen. The baby is arching and crying. Maria's hands are clenched around the baby, her jaw tight, her breathing is constricted, as if she herself is feeling the apparent belly pain that the little baby is experiencing. This level of body empathy is making it hard for Maria to comfort the baby.

Because she is so tight, she holds the baby out away from her body while her eyes fix on his face as she grimaces along with him. Within two minutes, the baby vomits, making it clear that Maria has not been exaggerating: the vomit spews across the room, the baby looks surprised and slightly relieved, and the mother shocked, overwhelmed, and apologetic.

After we tidy up a bit, Maria resettles into the rocking chair, baby in her arms. In this moment when he is less distressed, her body is markedly softer, less tense, and her breathing deepens. This combination of events then makes it possible for the baby to soften further. He settles in, more connected to her torso, and she shifts him in her arms, cuddling him.

She turns to me, worry spreading over her face. "It's going to happen again," she says, distraught. "He's going to do it again, and I don't know what to do."

I nod. "Well, maybe," I agreed, "but just notice what is happening now. Your arms are relaxed, and your breath is deeper." She takes a deep breath without prompting. "How is he doing right now?"

She looks at the baby. "Yes, better," she acknowledges. I can see her jaw soften slightly. She pulls him snugly into her. "Poor little baby, what a hard beginning."

"See how it is to hold him with your arms soft like that?" I offer. "He seems to like it. Do you like it?"

She looks up, almost smiling. "I just worry about what is going to happen and why this is happening and whether I can take much more." Her jaw tightens again with those words.

"Yeah," I say, blowing out a big breath (which I hope she'll mirror). "I know it's a worry. But this moment right now, this is a pretty nice moment." She considers that for a bit and then nods, actually smiling at the baby's face.

The pediatrician later confirms pyloric stenosis, a treatable condition. Having a diagnosis helped Maria to believe that her baby's vomiting and crying were not her fault. Even though the baby continued to struggle for a few weeks, Maria was able to comfort him more confidently and more effectively because she could relax into the process of "being with."

Possibly the worst side effect of the negative thinking of perinatal mood disorders is preoccupation. The mother is preoccupied with thinking about what a bad mother she is or that her baby is going to die, or that she should never have had children, or whatever fresh hell her mind creates. This means that her attention is on her thinking and how bad it makes her feel.

All this thinking separates her from her body sensations. She believes she's feeling "bad," but when she can genuinely check with her body, she might find it's not as terrible as her mind suggested. When she can slow her mind enough to check in, breathe, ground, and notice what is happening in the moment, she can be more emotionally available to herself and thus to her baby.

Polyvagal babies

Mothers have a polyvagal ANS (see Chapter 3), but babies have it too. In fact, a lot of what we know about the function of the ventral vagal system (remember the "social engagement system") comes from studying parent-infant interaction. Again, the ventral vagal is the part of the ANS that keeps everything functioning, allows us to connect to other mammals, and helps regulate our sympathetic arousal. The dance of interaction between mothers and babies is really a dance between two autonomic nervous systems. That might not sound very poetic, but it is a biological reality.

Maternal behaviors directed at infants stimulate the ventral vagal through soothing, feeding, and comforting—the spontaneous, everyday actions of baby care. Gently stroking the baby's cheek, as breastfeeding mothers do to stimulate the head-turning and mouth-opening reflex, also stimulates the ventral vagus. The gasping cry of hunger turns to sucking as the mother introduces the nipple. The action of sucking activates the ventral vagus, giving way to deeper, more relaxed breathing. Mother cradles the head, speaks softly into the ear, uses her high-pitched "motherese" voice, and all of these help calm the baby. The baby fills up and falls asleep, blissed-out and milk-drunk. The mother's body is activated by the contact, the sucking, the hormone cascade of nursing, and even the ongoing contact of body against body, skin touching skin. Her ventral vagal system dances with that of the baby.

Feeding is not a necessary component to help babies settle into a dominant social engagement mode. Parents can hold with relaxed arms, breathing in a deep and relaxed way and staying as calm as possible. Side-to-side motion and humming or quiet singing are time-tested ways to soothe an infant, but they also serve to soothe the parent. It is almost impossible to hum or sing and hold your breath at the same time. Humming tends to lengthen the exhalation, which signals the ANS to quiet the sympathetic system and engage the ventral vagal. Then the baby can relax and interact. Parents use behaviors to help babies settle, but even without trying their bodies provide a regulating function. Co-regulation is not the practice of trying to settle another person by being calm yourself. It is what happens automatically, spontaneously, without volition.

We don't have to try to co-regulate. In fact, co-regulation goes two ways. The other person's level of regulation is relevant too. Imagine your partner comes home in great distress. How does your body respond to that? With a baby, we assume they have little capacity for self-regulation, and so we are willing to take on more responsibility than we are for an adult, but our bodies do respond to the arousal/agitation of other adults. Similarly, we respond to the calmness exuded by another person.

Babies are clear when things are not okay; they let us know. It can be hard to stay calm when the baby is screaming, but a mother only has to stay calmer than the baby. That is, calm is not a binary either-or category but rather a matter of degree. A mother who is extremely distraught while her baby is distraught need only be slightly calmer than her child. The perfectionism of distressed thinking isn't helpful here. She doesn't have to be perfect, just a little calmer than her child.

The baby gets information from her body, much more than her words. How can her body tell the baby that everything is fine? While she holds the baby, she can relax her arms. Pressing her feet lightly into the ground will help her feel her whole body. She can settle into her chair a little more deeply and let out a sigh. Softening her face and jaw, she can speak kindly to herself, remind herself that she can be here, now, and with the baby, and that this moment of baby screaming will not last forever, however much it may feel that way in the moment.

Babies ground into their mothers' bodies

More than calming signals get communicated to infants. The body of the parent helps the baby organize himself. The parent's ANS provides information continuously to the baby's ANS, and at the same time, the parent provides stimulation in the forms of touch, pressure, movement, talking and singing, and the smells and tastes of the body. Obviously, we don't think a lot about these things, and sharing this information happens automatically and mostly unconsciously.

We know that babies as young as a day or two will prefer the scent of their mother's breast pad over another woman's scent, prefer their caregiver's handling as early as three to four months, and recognize their mothers' voices immediately after birth. These findings are the result of information shared between mother and baby.

Mothers also quickly learn about their babies and can recognize them by smell after only a brief period of contact. Biology sets us up to connect with our progeny and for babies to use their parents to support their development in both subtle and overt ways.

This makes sense. Newborn humans are peculiarly unable to survive without adult care, and so nature supplies them with a built-in way to get that adult care. They evoke a caregiving response in adults. Women who have given birth are flooded with connection hormones that predispose them to seek out their baby. The infant, for his part, uses reflexive movement to crawl up to her nipple and latch on. The flow of colostrum and then milk is an oxytocin-based release in the maternal body that generally feels very good. The warm body connection between baby and mother supports an ongoing system of care.

Part of the necessary care of newborn humans involves being carried, held, and supported while muscular and neurological development proceeds. Babies learn the edges and contours of their bodies by pushing and pressing into their parents. They stretch their legs and push their feet into their mothers' bellies and press their heads into their mothers' necks. Parents, in turn, feed, carry, undress, wash, dress, talk to their babies, and show them the world.

During his first year, when the infant learns to crawl, walk, understand and use some language, delay gratification a tiny bit, recognize and prefer family to strangers, and interact with adults, his mother, in particular, helps the baby develop into a human being.

Helping the baby feel his body becomes more important as he gets older, of course. Body play is a lovely and enjoyable part of baby care. Mothers and others play with the baby's toes, blow raspberries into fat bellies, and often perform ridiculous feats on repeat, if the baby laughs with pleasure.

Encouraging the baby to press with feet into the floor, or into your hands while he is lying on his back, helps him to feel where his body is in space. This kind of play, along with being carried, swung, and rocked, helps to develop both his vestibular senses and his experience of being in an autonomous body.

The body of the mother continues to grow the baby well after birth.

CHAPTER 16

Taking Care of the Therapist

What is your why?

You probably have an implicit reason for choosing perinatal work as well as an explicit one. You might "know" you're a perinatal therapist because of your own perinatal history, for example. But taking time to dig deep might yield more treasure. Excavating your own insides to shine light on your deepest desires as a therapist can help you stay the course when things get hard.

You sit in the therapy room with your clients, because you feel a call to do this work. There is something that makes the struggles of motherhood intensely interesting. For each therapist, there is some deeply personal reason why it matters.

The work is challenging, interesting, and important. It is also difficult. This is not a job where you can phone it in on a bad day. These clients call for the best of you. It can help, when you're exhausted, feeling overwhelmed, or flooded with client suffering, to remember your "why." It helps you return to the room, week after week, even when progress is slow or seems impossible.

You can also use your "why" to remind you to take care of yourself, and that's what this chapter is about.

I have learned to dislike the term "self-care." Like so many other useful phrases, it has been co-opted, but when I first heard it, the context was women who would not or could not take time to put on their own oxygen masks before trying to help everyone else. We're still stuck, at times, with the cultural expectations of women, and mothers in particular, to be self-sacrificing. But like anything, that can go too far. Everyone needs care. Everyone, including therapists.

Identifying your very personal "why" helps you care for yourself on every level. If you have a clear understanding of why this work is important to you, you will attend to your own needs so you can continue it. Defining your worth at work helps you feel your value in other places. When you can feel your value, simple care for your physical needs becomes obvious. You take a break, have a snack, go for a walk. Rest when tired.

If your "why" needs clarification, this exercise may help.

Exercise #47: (FOR THE THERAPIST) My Ideal Client

This is a journaling exercise that activates your imagination.

A. Imagine the client you are meant to work with. This might be the person you think about when you take training, read a book like this one, or talk with colleagues about your life's work. Give this client lots of details in your imagination. What is the age? The background? Perinatal status? What issues are presenting? Does she have a dog? Get along with her in-laws? Don't waffle with generalizations, but turn this idea into a very real person, like a character in a show.

As you develop your ideas, write about your client, paying attention to your own body sensations as you think about and describe her.

Feel the sensations in yourself as you think about your interactions with your imaginary ideal. Use one side of the paper for your description of your client and the other to make notes about what you notice as you think and write. The following prompts might be helpful, but you can also just write freely about this.

- Who is your client?
- What do you see when you look at her?
- What does she bring into your practice and your life?
- What do you honor about her coming to you?
- What are the gifts you give in therapy?
- What are the gifts you receive in therapy?

Notice when you feel like this writing session is over. You may or may not have completed this project, but you'll know. Maybe you have enough from one writing session. Perhaps you'll return to read over your pages and add some more.

B. Allow some time to lapse between A and B.

Read over your pages and notice what you feel and think. How does this client suit you now? As you read and notice, feel into why this client touches you and your work.

You can also ask this client (this imaginary person) why you are important to her. "Why did you choose me as your therapist?" Write down the answers that arise. Note if any of them seem to be filtered through a self-critical lens and let those go. From the answer or answers, you may be able to understand your motivation more clearly.

Social expectations and setting limits

If you are in the same stage of life as your clients, you may be dealing with similar issues at home and at work. Even if you're in a different life space, what you carry for your clients can sometimes feel very heavy.

As mentioned above, societal expectations for women, especially women who are mothers, include caring for everyone, often putting others' needs ahead of their own. There's a lot you could say about this injustice, but the mothers in your practice are probably facing expectations like these and may have internalized them. Mothers often struggle to acknowledge their needs while simultaneously carrying awareness of the needs of their children, partner, and members of the extended family. I've alluded to this earlier, but what's relevant here is whether those models of self-sacrifice, unfettered giving, and generosity of spirit are also informing your therapy practice.

Despite the idealization of selfless giving, it's not healthy when it results in depletion, depression or anxiety. The abnegation of self as practiced and encouraged in our cultural images of motherhood doesn't serve the mother. Similarly, it does not serve the therapist.

Mothers who are suffering need a lot from you. It's important for you to have a clear understanding of where your boundaries lie and how you will hold them in the face of this great need. Your thoughts about this will change as your own life changes. For example, if you have small children at home, your availability may be different from when your children are teens.

Finding and holding boundaries in the face of great need, as a perinatal therapist must, parallels the process mothers experience with their infants. During the first six months after birth, mothers are negotiating their sense of self-as-mother. Who am I now? Has this new baby changed me in some fundamental way? Much of the work of adaptation, within and outside therapy, is involved with her finding her feet again, locating the solid ground of being.

Helping clients with this requires you to have your own very solid ground of being, and that includes knowing your limits and where you can expand into meeting someone's needs. Don't ignore your inner sense that tells you when someone is asking too much of you. It might be true.

Doing the boundary exercises (see Chapter 11) while you are feeling activated about a client's demands can help you clarify where you want to set your limits and where you are willing to engage. You are a big support to clients. At the same time, you are not meant to be their only support.

Setting limits not only takes care of your needs but models a sustainable way to be. When clients see you setting limits on your work hours, being clear about your availability, and prioritizing your own care, it makes it more possible for them to make similar choices. Here you are, a respectable professional who is very helpful, and you model respect for yourself and your needs. It can be done.

Taking care of yourself is also caring for your clients in a more concrete way. When your needs are met, you are more available to clients. It is worthwhile to reflect on your practice, checking in to see if your work life is meeting your needs. For me, the number of appointments I have in a week makes a difference to my energy level. My capacity for presence drops when I see too many people. It's been a lesson for me: am I actually helping if I take another client, even knowing I won't have the energy for them? It's hard to say no to a need, but when I don't, I'm not as helpful to any of my clients.

This has taken me a long time to learn.

Going from depleted to recharged

Do you know when you're depleted?

Can you tell you're tired before you completely exhaust yourself? This is a skill, and if you typically try to fit too much into a day, you might not even realize when you are starting to need rest. Missing cues to rest can lead to burnout over time, so it's worthwhile to orient yourself to how your body feels when you need something.

Are you irritable? That's a clue. Something is not quite right. Keep checking in. Are you hungry, angry, lonely, tired?

If you can identify the need, you can take steps to meet it. Perhaps you've been sitting too long or staring at clients on a screen. Using your body awareness, ask your somatic self what you need right now.

Practice letting yourself have what you need, even if you can't have as much as you want. For example, you might desperately need an hour nap but you only have ten minutes before your next client. You could lie on the floor in constructive rest, letting your shoulders drop, feeling your weight sink into the earth, and letting ease into your joints. Or you might need a meal, but a snack could help take the edge off.

Make a note of what helps and how you notice a change. It can be a mental note, just to jog your memory. Next time you are irritable, what does your body need?

Too many people think "recharging" requires a week of vacation at a resort. Of course it might be a good recharge, but it's not available to most of us at the frequency we need to bolster our batteries. Don't forgo vacations but choose to insert sensory pleasures into every single day.

It may take time to learn what sensory delights feed your body and soul, but finding out is important. Notice pleasure arising in your day. Those moments are the juicy part of life and can come from almost anything—a bunch of tulips, a baby's giggle, steaming tea, the sun slanting onto your desk. Give yourself permission to really soak in the sensory experience. Savor it. Drink it in. It's for you, right now. Don't take a picture of it; be IN it.

When you've compiled a list of things that tickle your delight, arrange to have more of them. Set yourself up to enjoy moments in every day. When you experience them, lean in. Make sure you are fully present, body and mind. Make a note. What does your body enjoy that you can offer it regularly? How does your body respond to that?

That's a prescription for living your life right now. Use your somatic tools for your own good.

Exercise #48: (FOR THE THERAPIST) Somatic Discharge of Work-Related Stress

Working as a therapist is difficult and challenging and of course you love it. Some days are hard, though, and you can take home stress and distress. Use the tools you have learned to give yourself grace those days.

Begin in the orienting position. Press your feet into the ground and coordinate your breathing so that you bend your knees to inhale and exhale as you straighten your legs (but don't lock your knees). Keep on pushing the floor and breathing and paying attention to your body.

Now think about what you are bringing from work. Sometimes you bring home worry about a client, or frustration with them. These are your emotions. You are responsible for handling them. It is critical to get your feelings about clients sorted out so you're not inadvertently using clients to help you feel better. It also helps to prevent therapist burnout.

Notice what comes up. How does your body want to express that?

Here is an example: Perhaps your client cannot seem to take any action on her own behalf. Or maybe you are suffering along with your client, frustrated that those painful things are not changing. This exercise is about allowing for an expression of frustration.

Throw your elbows back, saying, "Get off my back" (see Chapter 14). Throw some pillows, hard. Pound a pillow with your fists, narrowing your eyes and sticking out your jaw. Pick one exercise and stay with it for a few minutes.

You can vocalize whatever you're carrying around. Remember that your words are just a container for the energy, so say whatever works.

"Stop it!" "We'll do it my way!" "No! I won't listen to you anymore!" Your clients are not hearing what you are saying, and it doesn't make you a bad therapist to discharge your feelings of frustration.

Notice your energy building and discharging. Feel into your body as your energy rises. Hold the container for it, let it build, then let the discharge happen (perhaps pitching your pillows ever harder).

Had enough? Before you simply stop the movement, try this. Do it a couple more times along with a loud protest. "I'm done! I don't want to! No more!" When you have protested and really felt the protest, then allow yourself to stop. Practicing your protest helps you keep good boundaries.

Return to the orienting position and take a breath. What was that like for you? What do you notice?

Welcome whatever you feel. There may be a few different feelings flowing around.

If your body wants more, try the exercise again. It is often useful to do an exercise three times and notice what changes. Check in to see how you are feeling about work after you have finished the exercise.

Sticky trauma

When you've been helping clients process trauma, you might find some of it feels "sticky." Releasing traumatic material is important, and an active discharge exercise such as throwing pillows ("This isn't mine") can help to get it out of your immediate sensory experience. The exercise above is also a good way to shift the energy of sticky trauma, particularly to clarify the boundaries.

Using your arms to push it away can help. Press the large yoga ball into the wall and push, push, push. Vocalize your desire. Then check in and see what has changed.

You can also try washing your hands in an intentional way, sluicing sticky trauma off your fingers and watching it slide down the drain. A room-clearing spray can also help you to limit the lingering effects of stress-inducing material. The shaking exercise from Chapter 12 helps here too.

If your own trauma gets activated by a client's work, implement self-care immediately, plus seek out support. That can be a chat with a colleague. If you don't find some settling and relief, consider supervision or consultation around that client. Getting activated isn't a problem in itself. The challenge lies in giving yourself enough time, space, and care to be able to care for your clients.

It is hard enough to work with your clients when you're feeling well. Calling your therapist, getting support from peers, and actively working on separating your material from that of the client are all helpful. In some cases, referring a client to another therapist is best for both of you, but it doesn't have to be the first step.

By working through this book, you've developed many tools for your practice. You can also use these tools to stay connected to yourself and to release frustration and prevent burnout. Here are the skills you've practiced. You can . . .

- Create a holding space in which bodies and minds are welcome as they are
- Model compassionate curiosity about the body-mind process
- Invite and accompany clients into their somatic experience
- Track somatic energy, your own and your clients'
- Experience your body resonance as a source of information
- Use breath to soften rigidity and ease suffering
- Support your clients' ANS regulation
- Assess grounding, plus teach and model increasing groundedness and support grounding
- Mirror and attune to somatic cues to both increase relating and enhance body resonance
- Explore and strengthen body-based boundaries
- Use movement to experience the here-and-now
- Express emotion directly through the body

- Support the parent-infant "dance" of relating, co-regulation, and development

That's a substantial list of skills that you can integrate with the therapies you offer. Using them yourself will support your self-care as you increase grounding, self-awareness, and self-possession.

Last words

The work you've undertaken is important work. Helping women to take the mantle of maternal identity in a way that genuinely honors the individual is significant. Your commitment reflects a multi-generational, cross-cultural tradition of women supporting women into and through motherhood. As a perinatal therapist, you are connected to ancestral caregivers back many generations. Even though you work with the newest methods and empirically supported interventions, and even though motherhood may look very discrepant from person to person and time to time, you are helping women to become mothers, just as many have done before you.

The person who gives birth to the baby often seems to disappear in the rush of interest in the new infant. Perinatal therapists keep our eyes firmly on the mother, and she is the locus of our work, and yet there is an element of the future in perinatal therapy that can make it ever more meaningful. The tiny changes that happen at the beginning of family life can lead to large differences in outcome.

When a woman feels capable and supported, she'll behave differently with her partner, her children and the new baby than if she feels anxious, stressed, incompetent, and isolated. It's not hard to guess which is better for her and better for her children. Even though our clients are much more than "just mothers," the work you do with them is grounded in the expectation that things can and will be better. Explicitly or implicitly, working with mothers is about creating a good future for them and their children. This is a profoundly hopeful stance to take in a world that can feel full of despair.

One of my greatest pleasures has been consultation with perinatal therapists. In these professional relationships, I've found people who are passionate about their work; focused on best practices within a flexible, compassionate supportive framework; and who collaborate and consult, supporting other therapists to do their best work while sharing ideas, resources, and help.

You are thoughtful, careful, and self-reflective. You bring a level of emotional maturity to this work that you may not even be aware of. You are humble, learning from your clients every day. I wish you all the best in your work with perinatal clients. Keep doing what you do: learning, sharing, listening, being with, growing.

Glossary

Adjustment period postpartum

For psychosocial/clinical purposes, the first year after the birth of a child comprises the postpartum period. In the medical arena, a woman is considered to be through her postpartum period at six weeks after the birth, though recovery from pregnancy and childbirth can take longer. Certainly, adjusting to having a new baby is an ongoing process.

Attachment history

The quality of the attachment between parent and infant predicts a variety of outcomes in childhood and even into adulthood. Securely attached infants tend to protest when separated from their attachment figure. Upon reunion, they may cry and reconnect but will readily return to playing, suggesting some level of comfort has been gained. Other attachment styles include avoidant, where the child barely attends to the parent's absence or return, and anxious, in which the distraught child cannot be soothed and cannot return to play upon the parent's return. A fourth category of attachment, disorganized, is seen in children with highly unpredictable social environments. Their behavior on separation and reunion is uncategorizable.

Early experiences that result in various types of parent-infant attachment result in patterns of expectations around relationships in general. Broadly speaking, a securely attached person will expect people to be predictable, reliable, and connected. Anxiously attached people may require closeness to make simple decisions, while avoidant folks become extremely independent and struggle with letting others help them.

Therapists' awareness of their personal attachment history is helpful when working with mothers and their infants. Otherwise, biases and expectations that are just beyond awareness can influence the work, perhaps in negative ways.

Autonomic nervous system (ANS)

The ANS is the part of the peripheral nervous system (spinal cord and nerves) that controls automatic functioning of the body. It is composed of the sympathetic and parasympathetic systems.

Autonomic arousal refers to activation of the sympathetic system, generally referred to as the "fight, flight, or freeze" system, because one of those three responses commonly occurs when arousal is heightened. Sympathetic arousal is not sexual arousal, though there is a sympathetic component in sexual arousal.

Autonomic reactivity refers to how quickly arousal can rise and fall. A person who is more reactive is likely to become aroused quickly and calm more slowly than a less reactive person.

Bioenergetic analysis

This form of body-oriented psychoanalysis was created by Alexander Lowen and John Pierrakos, after work with Wilhelm Reich in the USA in the 1950s and 1960s. Bioenergetic analysis differed from psychoanalysis by limiting interpretation of dreams, free association, and so forth to emphasize direct experience. The current forms of bioenergetic therapy are best represented by the International Institute for Bioenergetic Analysis in Barcelona, Spain.

Bioenergetic psychotherapy

Bioenergetic psychotherapy is the type of therapy currently practiced by many bioenergetic therapists who do not identify as analysts.

Body resonance (somatic resonance)

Human bodies are attuned to other bodies that share the same space. If a highly distressed person enters a group, other members of the group may begin to feel uncomfortable as their bodies resonate to that distress. This is a useful phenomenon in body psychotherapy, to the degree that the therapist is aware of how their body may be responding to the client.

Boundary wounding

When a person's psychological or somatic boundary has been violated, it may be felt as a wounded place. Similar to falling and scraping a knee, the transgression of a limit can create dysregulation and distress.

Cognitive behavioral therapy (CBT)

CBT is a type of talk psychotherapy in which negative patterns of thoughts about the self and the world are challenged. Goals include changing behavior patterns and treating disorders.

Co-regulation

Bodies spontaneously regulate one another when in the same place, due to the autonomic nervous systems communicating through the senses. One can observe co-regulation readily when looking at parent-infant interaction. The parent's body soothes the infant's body not only by behavior but through this unconscious mechanism.

Dorsal vagal

In the polyvagal theory, the dorsal vagal branch is the part of the vagus nerve of the parasympathetic nervous system that slows heart function, breathing, and facilitates digestion. The contrast is to the ventral vagal branch which includes connections with the ears, throat, face, and upper chest.

Dysregulated

When body systems are not operating in synchrony, a person may feel scattered or spacy. Dysregulation also reflects extremely high levels of sympathetic activation, as in fear or rage.

Ego-dystonic

When thoughts and feelings are inconsistent with a person's expectations of themselves, they are ego-dystonic. Intrusive thoughts that mothers experience in the postpartum period are common. When a mother is shocked or horrified by the intrusive image of harm to her baby, the thought is ego-dystonic, inconsistent with her sense of self. This ego-dystonia means she can separate herself from the thought. Identification of ego-dystonia helps distinguish between intrusive thoughts and those that represent a break from reality and require crisis intervention.

Ego-syntonic

Ego-syntonic thoughts and feelings are consistent with one's expectations for oneself. If thoughts of harming self and others seem normal and reasonable, they are ego-syntonic. When the thoughts do not reflect reality, such as when a mother imagines holding her baby under the bathwater to protect him from harm, there may be a psychotic process occurring.

Embodiment

The overtly physical sense of being an organic living person is embodiment. A contrast point is dissociation, or "feeling out of my body," which people sometimes say when they have been thinking too much, especially if the thoughts are painful. Attention to body sensations can help a person feel more embodied.

In other use, embodiment refers to engaging in behaviors and practices that "embody" some concept, such as "a good mother."

EMDR

Eye-movement desensitization and reprocessing (EMDR) is based on the idea that humans heal from traumatic injuries spontaneously but sometimes create obstacles that need to be removed. EMDR creates a setting where a client approaches the traumatic memory, along with the thoughts and body sensations, in a structured, supported way. This exposure desensitizes the person to the memory, thoughts, sensations, and feelings, and makes room for reinterpretation.

Emotional granularity

The more emotion labels we have, the broader and more satisfying our emotional experience, according to Lisa Feldman Barrett, PhD. Emotional granularity involves increasing the differentiation of emotions from a global categorization (happy, sad, angry, afraid) to include a wide variety of experiences of each.

Emotion-focused therapy

EFT is a type of psychotherapy that takes into account a person's attachment history and how their feelings are implicated in their thinking and behavior.

Implicit memory

Explicit memory includes everything we remember. Implicit memory includes things we remember but can't access directly. This example helped me understand the difference. A girl was brought to the hospital without recollection of her name, address, or phone number (this was back when people had to remember their numbers). When handed the phone, she was able to dial her mother's number. She had implicit memory for that number, at least when she was asked to enact a motor activity. But she could not recall it through verbal means.

In parenting young children, people often operate on implicit memory from their own infant and toddler experiences. Those experiences happened at too young an age to be remembered in words but reside in implicit memory. People "automatically know" how to parent, but the behaviors are based on implicit memory.

Interoception

Beyond the five senses of sight, hearing, smell, touch, and taste, there is interoception, which is a sense of what's going on inside the body physically and/or emotionally. Much of body-oriented psychotherapy is focused on helping clients pay attention to interoception.

Interpersonal therapy (IPT)

ITP is a form of psychotherapy that deals with the roles we take on such as family member, parent, worker, or adult caregiver. There is some evidence of IPT being useful for postpartum depression.

Maternal healing

This phrase, coined by Helena Vissing, Ph.D., reflects a focus on helping mothers in the mother-infant dyad of the postpartum during their recovery from the challenges of the perinatal period. See Resources for Vissing's book.

Maternal psychotherapy

Maternal psychotherapy is specifically oriented to women's issues of reproductive health. It can include decision-making about children, fertility issues, pregnancy and birth concerns, and postpartum well-being. It can go beyond the perinatal period to address mood and anxiety disorders, parenting, relationship, and other issues relevant to maternal identity.

Neuroception

Before we see or hear anything that might be "dangerous," our brains are on the job. Neuroception is a preconscious assessment that theoretically happens at the level of the brainstem. If a stimulus is "dangerous" the sympathetic nervous system alerts.

Normative process

Any process that most people go through during the course of development.

Parasympathetic nervous system (PNS)

The PNS is the branch of the autonomic nervous system that regulates homeostatic functions in the body as well as social connections via sight, sound, and touch, particularly around the face. It slows heart rate, increases respiration, lowers blood pressure, and supports elimination of waste.

Perinatal development

The baby isn't the only one developing throughout pregnancy and the first year after birth. Mothers, too, develop. Perinatal development, when applied to the mother, refers to the processes of change from the initial thinking about children, through achieving pregnancy, childbirth, and the first year of parenting.

Perinatal mental health work

Psychoeducation, counseling, psychotherapy, case management, or support groups related to childbearing and parenting infants are all examples of perinatal mental health work.

Perinatal psychotherapy

This term refers to psychotherapy that is undertaken during the perinatal period to address issues arising from reproductive experiences.

PMADs

This acronym means Perinatal Mood and Anxiety Disorders. These include diagnoses of adjustment disorder, depression, bipolar disorder, generalized anxiety, panic disorder, or obsessive-compulsive disorder, or post-traumatic stress disorder specific to the perinatal period and related to childbearing or child-rearing. PMADs do not include perinatal psychosis.

Polyvagal theory

The polyvagal theory was created by Stephen Porges and popularized for psychotherapy by Deb Dana. It's a conceptualization of the mammalian parasympathetic nervous system as comprised of two parts with distinct functions. The arms of the vagus nerves that innervate the front of the body help the person become available for social engagement, while the vagus nerves that innervate the back body are involved in moderating arousal, managing respiration, heart functions, and digestion. See Resources for a list of titles.

Postpartum

Postpartum refers to the recovery period after childbirth. Medically, it refers to six weeks after birth.

Process-oriented therapy

Process-oriented therapy focuses on the here-and-now experience rather than problem-solving or thinking. It often includes experiential components as well as talking.

Psychological defenses

Defenses are unconsciously enacted patterns of behavior and/or thinking that protect a person from anxiety. In the theory of bioenergetic analysis, childhood experiences of repeated distress result in characteristic holding patterns in the body. For example, a boy repeatedly shamed for crying will tighten his throat, stiffen his shoulders, and breathe shallowly to cut off crying and the associated emotion. These muscular holding patterns become chronic and result in body shapes that are predictive of behavioral defenses, according to Alexander Lowen. In this way, typical defenses are structured into the body. Lowen refers to patterns of defenses as character structure. For more information, see Lowen's books in Resources.

Psychosocial

Most influences on people arise from both their internal attributions and thoughts and the external world. The term psychosocial encompasses the internal and external plus the interaction of those influences.

PTSD

This acronym stands for Post-Traumatic Stress Disorder. This disorder, as defined by the Diagnostic and Statistical Manual of Mental Disorders by the American Psychiatric Association, has specific criteria. However, the term tends to be in broad use, albeit inaccurately, to refer to any kind of negative outcome from traumatic experiences.

Somatic

Anything relating to the body.

Somatic interventions

In psychotherapy, somatic interventions include suggested activities for clients that are specifically oriented to physical experience.

Somatic memory

Memory experienced as a feeling or sensation in the body rather than as a story is a somatic memory. Often it will be connected to a story or image.

Somatic psychotherapy

Somatic psychotherapy prioritizes a person's experiences over their thoughts. It will usually use body-based interventions such as movement or a focus on breathing to access psychological material.

Sympathetic nervous system

The sympathetic nervous system is the branch of the autonomic nervous system that is responsible for activating the "fight, flight, or freeze" response when danger is anticipated or present. It also helps increase heart rate, supports immune function, regulates blood glucose levels, and affects gut motility. It tends to have an activating function.

Titration

Titration is a process of gradually exposing someone to a stimulus to find the optimal level to achieve a particular goal. In trauma therapy, we titrate exposure to disturbing stimuli as clients increase their tolerance.

Traumatic stress

Challenging events can cause an extreme response in the body that does not resolve spontaneously within a day or so. People find different things stressful and individual tolerance for stress varies. The heightened sensitivity of perinatal clients is a factor in how they manage stressors. Traumatic stress refers to the pattern of sleep disturbances, avoidance, and reexperiencing that can occur when the body has been extremely stressed.

Ventral vagal nerve

In the "polyvagal theory," the ventral vagal nerve, in the front of the body, includes branches connecting to the ears, throat, face, and upper chest, and is implicated in the social engagement system. In contrast, the dorsal vagal, in the back body, slows heart function, digestion, and breathing.

Vestibular

The vestibular system, part of our sensory system of perception, is activated by head movement. It's located in the inner ear, and as the orientation of the ear to the earth changes, we experience different sensations. It can be soothing to have repetitive vestibular stimulation, such as rocking. It can be activating or arousing to have irregular stimulation, as a child might experience if a parent were roughhousing with them.

Working model

We develop ideas about how the world operates based on our experiences, thus creating an internal model for our world. The model is modifiable, based on new experiences. The early attachment researchers used "working model" to refer to the ideas young children build up about how relationships work. For example, a baby who experiences responsive parenting has a working model of a responsive world.

Bibliography

Barrett, Lisa F., and James A. Russell, eds. *The Psychological Construction of Emotion.* The Guilford Press, 2014.

Beck, C. T., and J. Driscoll. *Postpartum Mood and Anxiety Disorders: A Clinician's Guide.* Jones & Bartlett Learning, 2006.

Beck, C. T., J. W. Driscoll, and S. Watson. *Traumatic Childbirth.* Routledge, 2013.

Boyce, W. Thomas, Marla B. Sokolowski, and Gene E. Robinson. "Toward a new biology of social adversity." *Proceedings of the National Academy of Sciences* 109, Supplement 2 (2012):17143–17148.

Caldwell, Christine. *Bodyfulness: Somatic Practices for Presence, Empowerment, and Waking Up in This Life.* Shambhala, 2018.

Chin, Kathleen, Amelia Wendt, Ian M. Bennett, and Amritha Bhat. "Suicide and Maternal Mortality." *Curr Psychiatry Rep* 24 (2022):239–275. https://doi.org/10.1007/s11920-022-01334-3.

Covington, Sharon N., and Linda H. Burns, eds. *Infertility Counseling: A Comprehensive Handbook for Clinicians.* Cambridge University Press, 2006.

Dana, Deb. *The Polyvagal Theory in Therapy: Engaging the Rhythm of Regulation* (Norton Series on Interpersonal Neurobiology). W. W. Norton & Company, Inc., 2018.

Felitti, V. J. "Childhood sexual abuse, depression, and family dysfunction in adult obese patients: a case control study." *Southern Medical Journal* 86(7) (July 1993):732–736.

Fraiberg, Selma, Edna Adelson, and Vivian Shapiro. "Ghosts in the Nursery: A Psychoanalytic Approach to the Problems of Impaired Infant-Mother Relationships." *Journal of American Academy of Child Psychiatry* 14(3) (2003):387–421.

Gendlin, Eugene T. *Focusing-Oriented Psychotherapy: A Manual of the Experiential Method.* New York: The Guilford Press, 1998.

Jaffe, Janet, and Martha O. Diamond. *Reproductive Trauma: Psychotherapy with Infertility and Pregnancy Loss Clients.* Washington, DC: American Psychological Association, 2011.

Kleiman, Karen. *Therapy and the Postpartum Woman: Notes on Healing Postpartum Depression for Clinicians and the Women Who Seek Their Help.* Routledge, Taylor & Francis Group, 2008.

Kleiman, Karen. *The Art of Holding in Therapy: An Essential Intervention for Postpartum Depression and Anxiety.* Routledge, Taylor & Francis Group, 2017.

Kleiman, Karen, and Amy Wenzel. "Principles of supportive psychotherapy for perinatal distress." *Journal of Obstetric, Gynecologic & Neonatal Nursing* 46(6) (November–December 2017):895–903.

Levine, Peter A., and Ann Frederick. *Waking the Tiger: Healing Trauma: The Innate Capacity to Transform Overwhelming Experiences.* Berkeley: North Atlantic Books, 1997.

Lieberman, Alicia F., Elena Padrón, Patricia Van Horn, and William W. Harris. "Angels in the nursery: The intergenerational transmission of benevolent parental influences." *Infant Mental Health Journal: Official Publication of The World Association for Infant Mental Health* 26(6) (November 2005):504–520.

Lowen, Alexander. *Bioenergetic: The Revolutionary Therapy That Uses the Language of the Body to Heal the Problems of the Mind.* Penguin Random House, 1975, 1994.

Lowen, Alexander. *The Way to Vibrant Health: A Manual of Bioenergetic Exercises.* Simon and Schuster, 1977, 2012.

Michel, Elizabeth. *Bent Out of Shape: Anatomy and Alignment for Bioenergetic Trainees.* Self-published, 1997.

Porges, Stephen W. *The Polyvagal Theory: Neurophysiological Foundations of Emotions, Attachment, Communication, and Self-Regulation* (Norton Series on Interpersonal Neurobiology). W. W. Norton & Company, 2011.

Powell, Bert, Glen Cooper, Kent Hoffman, and Bob Marvin. *The Circle of Security Intervention: Enhancing Attachment in Early Parent-Child Relationships.* The Guilford Press, 2013.

Rothschild, Babette. *The Body Remembers Volume 2: Revolutionizing Trauma Treatment.* W. W. Norton & Company, 2017.

Rothschild, Babette. Autonomic Nervous System Table: Laminated Card. W. W. Norton & Company, 2017.

Stern, Daniel N. *The Interpersonal World of the Infant: A View from Psychoanalysis and Developmental Psychology.* Routledge, 2018.

Stern, Daniel N. *The Motherhood Constellation: A Unified View of Parent-Infant Psychotherapy.* Routledge, 1998, 2019.

Ure, L. (in press). "What's the Use?: A Body/Mind Journey from the Despair of Depression to Living with Vitality."

Vissing, Helena. *Somatic Maternal Healing: Psychodynamic and Somatic Trauma Treatment for Perinatal Mental Health.* Routledge, 2024.

Wenzel, A., with Karen Kleiman. *Cognitive Behavioral Therapy for Perinatal Distress.* Routledge, 2014.

Resources

Postpartum Support International (PSI) offers training for therapists and psychoeducation and support for families. PSI also offers the first certification for perinatal mental health specialists.

Karen Kleiman's practice, **The Postpartum Stress Center**, offers therapy for individuals and training for advanced practice clinicians. Karen has written a hefty number of books on perinatal distress and perinatal therapy, and she is an active force in supporting developing clinicians as well as mothers.

The International Institute of Bioenergetic Analysis (IIBA) is the global center for training in Bioenergetic Analysis, the somatic psychotherapy that lies at the foundation of this book. The IIBA also publishes the *IIBA Journal*, a clinical journal for somatic practitioners.

The United States Association for Body Psychotherapy (USABP) is a good resource for various other therapies and training programs, regular webinars, and a rich database of articles. USABP also publishes a research journal, in collaboration with the European Association of Body Psychotherapists, that offers empirical support for somatic methods.

Circle of Security International has an online presence that offers helpful materials for parents around attachment and a list of trained facilitators for their programs. They also offer training in the COS-Parenting model, an empirically supported program that supports development of secure attachments between parent and child.

Your free, downloadable personal **somatic exercise journal** can be found at https://bookhip.com/FVSHJCN. It's in printable PDF format for ease of use.

www.ingramcontent.com/pod-product-compliance
Lightning Source LLC
Chambersburg PA
CBHW041951020426
42342CB00036B/119